An Introduction to
Inherited Metabolic Diseases

An Introduction to Inherited Metabolic Diseases

J.B. Holton
Pathology Department
Southmead General Hospital
Westbury-on-Trym
Bristol

LONDON   NEW YORK

Chapman and Hall

First published in 1985 by
Chapman and Hall Ltd
11 New Fetter Lane, London EC4P 4EE
Published in the USA by
Chapman and Hall
29 West 35th Street, New York NY 10001

© 1985 J.B. Holton

Printed in Great Britain by
J.W. Arrowsmith Ltd., Bristol

ISBN 0 412 25220 1

Library of Congress Cataloging in Publication Data

Holton, J. B. (John B.)
  An introduction to inherited metabolic diseases.

  Bibliography: p.
  Includes index.
  1. Metabolism, Inborn errors of.   I Title.
[DNLM: 1. Metabolism, Inborn Errors.   WD 205 H758i]
RC627.8.H65   1985   616.3'9   85–15187
ISBN 0–412–25220–1 (pbk.)

British Library Cataloguing in Publication Data

Holton, J.B.
  An introduction to inherited metabolic diseases.
  1. Metabolism, Inborn errors of
  I. Title
  616.3'9042   RC627.8

  ISBN 0–412–25220–1

Contents

Preface   vii

1   Diseases, enzymes and genes   1
1.1   Inborn errors of metabolism   1
1.2   Genes and enzymes   3
1.3   Modes of inheritance   4
1.4   The primary gene products   7

2   The nature of the defects in enzyme synthesis   9
2.1   Genetic control of protein synthesis   9
2.2   Structurally altered enzymes   13
2.3   Possible defects in the rate of enzyme synthesis   21

3   Genetic heterogeneity   24
3.1   Introduction   24
3.2   Enzyme variation in normal individuals   25
3.3   Genetic variation in disease states   30
3.4   Heterogeneity in the expression of an enzyme defect in different cell types   38
3.5   Variable enzyme expression in heterozygotes   41
3.6   Variations in clinical expression   45

4   Secondary biochemical consequences and pathogenic mechanisms in the inherited metabolic diseases   48
4.1   Introduction   48
4.2   Distribution of defects   49
4.3   Pathogenic mechanisms related to derangement of cellular metabolism   56
4.4   Disorders of membrane function   68

5   Diagnosis of inherited metabolic diseases   74
5.1   Introduction   74

5.2 General principles of biochemical diagnosis 75
5.3 Conventional diagnostic procedures 82
5.4 Newborn population screening 82
5.5 Prenatal diagnosis 84

Suggestions for further reading and for reference 94

Index 96

Preface

The purpose of this book is to describe concisely and systematically the principles involved in understanding and investigating human inherited metabolic diseases. Numerous examples of human genetic disorder and variation are included in the text to illustrate these principles and, in this way, most of the better known and more interesting conditions are mentioned. However, there is no intention to provide all the essential information on a comprehensive range of disorders. For this the reader should refer to one of the larger textbooks of inherited metabolic diseases.

The approach which is used here was formulated in a series of lectures which have been given to biochemistry students for a number of years, and the book is written primarily for the undergraduate. It assumes a very basic knowledge of physiology, biochemistry, classical genetics and molecular genetics. It is hoped that the student will see that much of what has been learned as pure science is directly relevant to human disease. It is possible that the brief descriptions of the diseases may contain a little unfamiliar medical or pathological terminology. Because of this, two medical dictionaries are listed in the bibliography.

The book should be of use also to many of those whose work requires them to have a knowledge of the inherited metabolic diseases; for example, clinical biochemists, medical laboratory scientific officers and clinicians, particularly paediatricians. It is hoped that they will acquire a deeper understanding of the fundamental basis of the diseases and that this will help them to interpret more fully and accurately the observations they make.

1

Diseases, enzymes and genes

1.1 Inborn errors of metabolism

The most important single development in human biochemical genetics was the introduction of the concept of inborn errors of metabolism at the beginning of this century by Archibald Garrod, a London physician. These ideas have been extended and refined but in their original form they remain a useful working hypothesis for the diagnosis and investigation of patients with these conditions. Garrod formulated his concept from studies of four biochemical disorders; namely, alkaptonuria, cystinuria, pentosuria and albinism.

People are usually discovered to have alkaptonuria because their urine darkens on standing in air. They excrete abnormally large quantities of homogentisic acid, a metabolite of phenylalanine and tyrosine, and this is oxidized under alkaline conditions to a black polymer which is called alkapton (Fig 1.1). The same pigment

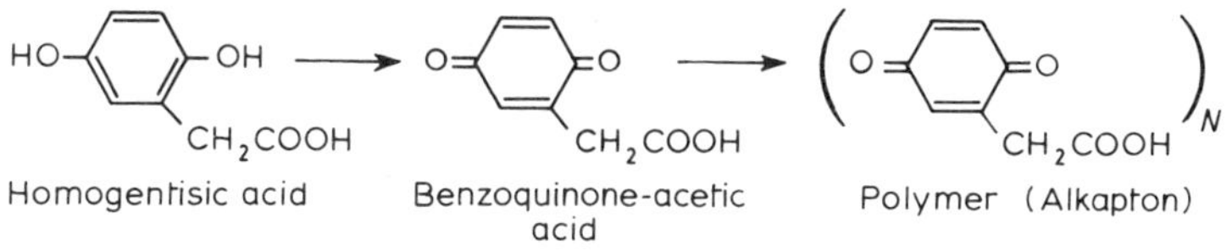

Homogentisic acid → Benzoquinone-acetic acid → Polymer (Alkapton)

Fig. 1.1 Formation of alkapton from homogentisic acid.

accumulates within the body of patients with the disorder, binding particularly to connective tissue; and may cause early degeneration of these tissues.

Pentosuria is mainly found by routine urine testing for diabetes mellitus. However, the reducing sugar which is excreted in excessive amounts is not glucose but the pentose xylulose, which is an intermediate in the pentose pathway of glucose oxidation. This particular biochemical abnormality does not appear to cause any disease symptoms.

Cystinuria is a cause of stone deposition in the urinary tract. Patients with the disease usually develop stones at an early age, often in the first decade of their life. They excrete an increased concentration of cystine, a relatively insoluble amino acid, and it crystallizes within the urinary tract. Garrod sought to explain this condition in terms of altered cystine metabolism but it was discovered after many years that it was a disorder of cystine transport. The precise mechanism of this defect will be looked at later.

The final disorder which attracted Garrod was albinism, a well-known condition which occurs in man and many animal species. There is a lack of normal dark pigmentation particularly in the hair, skin and eyes. The pigment which is absent is melanin, a substance which is normally synthesized from the amino acid tyrosine. This metabolic disorder will also be discussed more fully in a subsequent chapter.

Garrod reasoned that the four conditions shared two important features. Firstly, they were all 'inborn' or inherited. They tended to occur in several children in a family, but not in successive generations. In other words, they were examples of Mendelian recessive conditions. Secondly, they each demonstrated a marked chemical abnormality; in three a large excess of abnormal compound was excreted, in the other a normal body constituent could not be made. He did not have specific knowledge of the metabolism of the compounds he was interested in but he did see that the concept of the metabolic pathway, which had only recently been introduced, could be used to explain the chemical disorder.

The simple picture which emerged from Garrod's studies was that these inherited disorders could be explained by a block, or error, occurring in a metabolic pathway. A hypothetical pathway for the synthesis of D from its precursor A, through two intermediate compounds B and C is shown in Fig. 1.2(a). This could have a block occurring between C and D and one consequence would be that the end product D is not formed (Fig 1.2(b)), as for example the melanin in albinism. Also, the immediate precursor C will tend to accumulate and be excreted in abnormal amounts. Sometimes the other precursors (B, and A and B) may accumulate also (Fig. 1.2(c)), either because the steps in the pathway are reversible, or the increased concentration of C may inhibit the preceeding reactions. A further

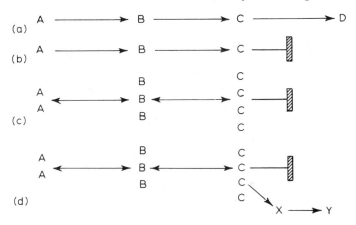

Fig. 1.2 (a)–(d)   The concept of the metabolic block and its consequences.

complication which we now know may occur, is metabolism of the excessive amounts of C along unusual pathways; thus a series of abnormal compounds (X and Y) may be formed and excreted (Fig. 1.2(d)).

Two other important points should be stressed about Garrod's work. Firstly, he stated that the metabolic block is the primary change and that when biochemical and disease changes occur they are all a secondary consequence of the block. In many diseases it has proved far more difficult to elucidate the mechanisms leading to the secondary events than to understand the fundamental defect itself. Secondly, in pentosuria, we had an example of a gross biochemical abnormality without any disease process occurring. Biochemical variation may be a normal phenomenon. Unfortunately, it is easy to forget that this can happen and a metabolic defect found in a patient may not necessarily be causally related to the disease signs and symptoms shown.

1.2   Genes and enzymes

Garrod's work pointed to the conclusion that the inheritance of certain metabolic diseases was determined by genes, following a simple Mendelian pattern. The idea that the primary cause of the biochemical changes, the metabolic block, is a defective enzyme was also contained in Garrod's original papers, but he is rarely credited with it. The working connection between genes and enzymes, or the one gene – one enzyme hypothesis, is attributed to Beadle and Tatum and was arrived at from a consideration of research on the fruit fly *Drosophila melanogaster* and the micro-organism *Neurospora crassa*.

It was possible to establish the relation between genes and biochemical processes with greater clarity by the experimental approach than by simple observations of human disorders, but Beadle and Tatum were the first to admit the foresight in Garrod's work.

Molecular genetics has now given us a much greater knowledge of the nature of genes, their enzyme products and the link between them. These ideas will be explored in subsequent chapters. It remains important, however, to consider the classical modes of inheritance of the metabolic conditions, particularly because it is often necessary to explain the risks of recurrence to affected families.

1.3 Modes of inheritance

Most metabolic disorders have autosomal recessive inheritance. This means that the individual who demonstrates the overt biochemical signs, and the associated disease picture if there is one, is homozygous for a mutant gene; that is they possess two altered genes instead of the normal genes which determine a particular enzyme. Usually the affected enzyme is almost completely inactive in such people. Both parents of a homozygous subject may be at least heterozygous, or carriers, for the condition, possessing one mutant gene and one normal gene. One, or both, parent could be homozygous for the mutant gene, but this rarely happens. In the typical situation, two heterozygous parents have a 1 in 4 chance of conceiving a homozygous abnormal child, the same chance of a homozygous normal child and a 2 in 4 chance of reproducing their own carrier genotype (Fig. 1.3). Thus, there is a 1 in 4 chance of producing a child with the disorder, but a three times greater chance of having a child who will be unaffected.

On looking more closely at the heterozygous individuals it becomes apparent that the conditions are not always strictly recessive. In simple terms, one would expect that they would have half the normal amount of enzyme, and this is often true. However, for reasons which will be explained in later chapters, heterozygotes may have more, or less, than 50% enzyme activity, in some cases it is much less. In many conditions it is possible to demonstrate the reduced enzyme

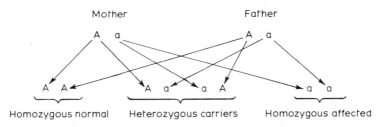

Fig. 1.3 Possible genotype of offspring in autosomal recessive inheritance: A, normal gene for a characteristic; a, mutant allelic form of the gene. Random association of the genes at conception results in three possible genotypes – AA, Aa and aa, the probability of each occurring being in the ratio 1: 2: 1 respectively.

activity in the heterozygotes and the secondary biochemical changes may even be present in a mild form. At the extreme end of this spectrum are conditions in which the biochemical manifestations in the heterozygote may approach, or may be indistinguishable from, the homozygous abnormal subject and they may show disease features. The disorder has then become *dominant* and the pattern of inheritance changes significantly. Only one parent is required to be heterozygous and may, of course, demonstrate all signs of the condition. There is a 50% chance of producing a similarly affected child (Fig. 1.4). In the unfortunate circumstance of both parents being heterozygotes there is a 3 in 4 chance of a child having the condition. Completely dominant conditions are quite rare, however.

The other mode of inheritance which is fairly common, having been demonstrated in well over 60 disorders, is X-linked recessive. In this case the enzyme which is defective is determined by a gene

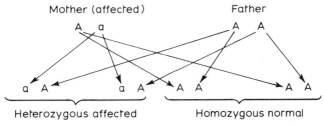

Fig. 1.4 Possible genotype of offspring in autosomal dominant inheritance. The designation of genes is the same as in Fig. 1.3. At conception there are two possible genotypes aA, these individuals being affected, and AA. The probability of each occurring is equal.

carried only on the X chromosome. Males are much more likely to be affected than females, having only a single X chromosome, but the disorder is transmitted principally through a female carrier, who is heterozygous for the abnormal gene. Male offspring have a 50% chance of being affected and female offspring a 50% chance of being heterozygous. Otherwise the children, both males and females, have a normal genotype with respect to the disorder (Fig. 1.5).

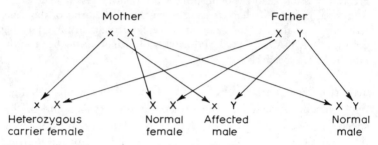

Fig. 1.5 Possible genotypes of the offspring in X-linked recessive inheritance. X and Y indicate the normal sex chromosomes and x a mutant X gene. Random association of the genes at conception results in the genotypes shown. There is a 1 in 4 chance of producing an affected male child and the same chance of a heterozygous carrier female.

It is a matter of some consequence in considering the enzyme expression of genes on the X chromosome, that although it would appear that normal females should have twice the amount of enzyme activity than normal males this is not usually the case. For most enzymes determined by genes on the X chromosome males and females have about the same normal range. The reason for this is explained by the Lyon hypothesis, which states that in any cell only one of the female's X chromosomes is actively expressed. It is postulated that at some stage in early embryological development random inactivation of one of the X chromosomes in each cell occurs, either that chromosome originating from the mother or that from the father. Clones of cells derived from each of these cells from then on perpetuate the particular X inactivation of the parent cell. Thus, in the heterozygous female, about half the cells may express the chromosome containing the normal gene and have normal enzyme activity; the others may express only the abnormal gene and have negligible enzyme activity. The mean activity of the two populations of cells is around 50% of normal. It is extremely interesting that 'Lyonization' does not occur with all enzymes determined by X-linked genes; for example, the enzyme steroid sulphatase, or placental sulphatase, normal females have almost twice as much enzyme activity as normal males.

Similarly to the situation described for conditions involving the autosomes heterozygotes for genes on the X chromosome may have very variable expression of the abnormal gene and, in extreme cases, may show marked biochemical and disease changes. The condition will then be seen as an X-linked dominant. However, it may be found that the disorder is expressed much more severely in males compared to heterozygous females, presumably reflecting quantitative differences in residual enzyme activity. In X-linked dominant conditions, if the mother is a heterozygote both male and female children have a 50% chance of being affected. If only the father carries the abnormal gene, female children will have a 50% chance of being affected, but the disorder cannot be inherited by the male children.

1.4 The primary gene products

The first genetic variations discovered mostly involved problems of enzyme synthesis which frequently give rise to very distinct biochemical and pathological changes. The study of human biochemical genetics now encompasses much wider aspects of molecular variation than this and primary gene products may be arbitrarily classified into proteins of two groups. Firstly, proteins concerned with transport of substances across membranes. Secondly, proteins circulating in the blood. It is probable that these represent only a small part of the total range of genetic variation because the scope of investigations in the human is severely limited.

The idea of a defect in membrane transport was first postulated in 1951 by Dent and Rose to explain their findings in the condition known as cystinuria, which was mentioned earlier in reference to Garrod's work. It was found that, in cystinuria, there was a large excess excretion not only of cystine, but of three other amino acids, ornithine, arginine and lysine. A common transport mechanism for all four amino acids, which was defective in cystinuria, could account for an observed decrease in absorption from the small intestine, and in reabsorption in the renal tubule. The poor renal tubular reabsorption, and not a defect in the metabolism, was shown to be the cause of increased urinary excretion of cystine. Since this first discovery, further disorders of amino acid transport mechanisms have been described and transport disorders for other substances, for example monosaccharides and inorganic ions. There is considerable evidence that the active transport systems involve specific proteins and that inherited defects in these proteins cause the transport disorders.

Numerous inherited disorders have been recognized involving abnormalities in blood proteins. The original function of the molecules affected in these disorders varies widely; it includes some which have a transporting role in the circulation (albumin, haemoglobin, lipoproteins), hormones (growth hormone and insulin), coagulation factors (Factors I to XIII), substances involved in immune systems (complement components and immunoglobulins) and enzyme inhibitors (a_1-antitrypsin and C_1 esterase inhibitors). There will be little systematic reference to these except to the disorders of haemoglobin synthesis which have contributed very much to our understanding of molecular defects.

The final area to return to is that of protein heterogeneity, or polymorphism, within the 'normal' population. It has already been mentioned that enzyme defects associated with gross secondary biochemical abnormalities may be consistent with complete clinical normality. In addition, it is now appreciated that there is much heterogeneity in the molecular structure of the enzymes within a population of individuals with normal enzyme activity. Typical examples of this phenomenon will be described in a later chapter.

2

The nature
of the defects in
enzyme synthesis

2.1 Genetic control of protein synthesis

2.1.1 Introduction

The first indication for the genetic control of protein synthesis arose from the study of human inherited metabolic diseases. It was difficult to obtain further insight into the mechanisms of this control, mainly because of the ethical constraints of experimentation on humans. However, molecular genetics has developed rapidly from work with insects and particularly micro-organisms. How far this work can be applied to mammalian cells is still not entirely clear, but certainly much of it is relevant and useful in the study of human disorders. Such attempts to understand the basic mechanisms of enzyme abnormality are not just of academic interest, but in many cases are an essential step to formulating logical methods of treatment.

2.1.2 Mechanism of genetic control of protein synthesis

The various stages in the expression of a gene are shown in Fig. 2.1. The genes themselves, which average about 1000 base pairs of a Watson-Crick double helix, consist of coding regions, or exons, which eventually determine the amino acid sequence of the protein product, interspersed with non-coding regions, called introns or intervening sequences (IVS). In addition, between the genes there are even larger lengths of spacer, or intergenic, DNA which are not transcribed. The whole purpose of the intergenic regions is unknown: however, to the left, or 'upstream', of the 5' end of the gene,

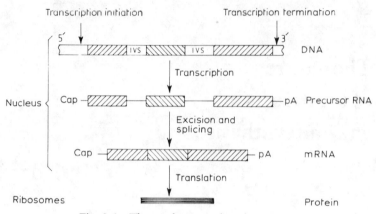

Fig. 2.1   The mechanism of gene expression.

there are a number of base sequences which are essential for initiating and for determining the rate of gene transcription.

Gene transcription proceeds from left to right, from the 5' to the 3' end of the DNA strand, reading both the exons and introns. This first product of gene expression is called precursor RNA and two other regular features of RNA are introduced at this stage. A 7-methylguanosine group is joined to the 5' terminal nucleotide through a 5'–5' pyrophosphate link. This grouping, called the Cap, is thought to enhance the efficiency of translation and it is common to all mammalian RNA molecules. Also, most RNAs have a tail of adenine molecules (pA) attached to the 3' terminal nucleotide. The significance of this addition in the post-translational region of the RNA molecule is unclear.

In the next stage, known as processing, non-coding lengths of nucleotides are excised from the precursor RNA and the coding portions are spliced together in a continuous sequence to yield processed, or messenger, RNA (mRNA). The portions of RNA which have to be removed during the processing are indicated by specific nucleotide sequences at the beginning and end of the IVS.

In the final step, mRNA is transported from the cell nucleus to the ribosomes where translation of the RNA code to the amino acid sequence of a specific protein occurs.

2.1.3   Disorders of gene expression

In the human, disorders of haemoglobin synthesis have been the most researched gene expression defects. These studies have demonstrated three principal forms of abnormality.

(1) Normal amounts of protein are synthesized, but it is structurally abnormal, having a substitution of one amino acid for another in its primary amino acid sequence. This is the nature of the variant forms of haemoglobin; the one amino acid substitution occurring in either the α-or β-globin chain of the normal haemoglobin molecule ($\alpha_2 \beta_2$). This type of abnormality is much more common in β globin.

(2) There is no detectable protein produced.

(3) Structurally normal protein is synthesized, but in significantly reduced quantities.

(2) and (3) are the basis of the conditions known as thalassaemias in which there is either a complete failure of synthesis of one of the globin chain types (α° or β° thalassaemia), or a reduced rate of production of the chains (α^+ or β^+ thalassaemia).

The first of the above defects is by far the most frequent of the haemoglobin disorders; the best-known variant, haemoglobin S, occurring in sickle cell disease. It is also likely that this is the most likely cause of abnormality in the synthesis of all proteins. It arises through a single base substitution in the coding portion of the gene and this is termed a point mutation. DNA transcription, RNA processing and translation all proceed at a normal rate, but the mRNA produced codes one amino acid wrongly in the primary sequence of the protein. In the sickle cell mutation there is a change from T to A at position 20 of the DNA of the β-gene on chromosome 11. In the corresponding mRNA sequence the triplet code for the amino acid at position 6 of the β-globin becomes GUG instead of GAG and this leads to a substitution of glutamic acid for valine at this site in the polypeptide chain.

The second type of defect can occur in a number of ways. Firstly, there may be a complete, or almost complete, deletion of the gene from the chromosome. For example in one severe type of α° thalassaemia, haemoglobin Bart's hydrops foetalis, both genes which code for the α-globin chain are lost in a massive deletion of bases from the short arm of chromosome 16. Secondly, even a small deletion or addition of bases, or a simple substitution in the nucleotide sequence of DNA, either in the intergenic region upstream to the gene or within the gene itself, may prevent the synthesis of any coherent mRNA. This may be because the signals to start transcribing the gene are lost, or because the specific splicing sequences in the IVS are altered in such a way that no normal mRNA can be processed from its precursor. Thirdly, in some cases of a small deletion or addition, or a substitution, the mRNA is synthesized at a normal rate, but the mutation produces a chain termination signal within the amino acid coding sequence. In these so-called nonsense mutations, polypeptide chain synthesis is terminated prematurely during the translation process and the truncated protein is usually destroyed rapidly within the cell. Finally, it is possible that regulator gene defects, similar to those found in micro-organisms, may occur in mammals. Although study of the thalassaemias suggest this is uncommon, it does not exclude it completely.

The third class of defect, in which reduced synthesis of a structurally normal protein occurs, may be caused by similar base deletions, additions or substitutions, as above, in which gene transcription, or normal precursor RNA processing, is affected, but not completely prevented. In these disorders, some normal mRNA is synthesized, and translated.

2.1.4 *Molecular mechanisms of the inherited metabolic diseases*

The circumstances which made possible the elucidation of the genetic mechanisms in the haemoglobin disorders, particularly the fairly easy availability of DNA, mRNA and protein for sequencing, do not exist in the case of the enzyme defects of the metabolic diseases. It has not been possible to study the disorder of gene expression in the enzyme defects in a direct way. It is not difficult, however, to obtain enough material to study the activity and characteristics of an enzyme, because this is a very sensitive property of these specific proteins. From these investigations it has been possible to make inference about the mechanism of the abnormality in quite a number of disorders.

Enzyme defects may be simply classified into those in which there is some residual enzyme activity and those in which there is none. The former of these could be caused by the synthesis of a structurally altered enzyme, or by a partial loss of ability to make the normal enzyme. It is usually possible to investigate these two possibilities by comparing the properties of the enzyme with those of the normal enzyme and in nearly all cases the structurally altered enzyme is the likely explanation. Examples of this will be discussed in the next section.

Metabolic disorders in which no activity of the relevant enzyme can be detected are much more difficult to investigate. Essentially, they could be due to a structural defect in the enzyme which impairs completely its catalytic activity, or by a total failure of protein synthesis. One line of study which has been pursued in this situation is to raise an antibody to the purified normal enzyme and to look for an antigenic reaction to the antibody, or for cross reacting material (CRM), in the blood or extracted tissues of a patient. In patients who show a reaction with the antigen (CRM positive), it must be assumed that a structurally similar protein to the normal enzyme is produced but that it is catalytically inactive. However, a CRM negative response could be due to a complete failure of enzyme synthesis, or to the production of a protein which is so altered that it no longer binds to the antibody to normal enzyme. Although the precise interpretation of these immunological studies may be difficult, it will be seen in a later chapter that the CRM concept is useful in demonstrating the heterogeneous nature of the enzyme defect in different patients with the same metabolic abnormality.

2.2 Structurally altered enzymes

As was stated in the previous section, it is possible in many defects with some residual enzyme activity to demonstrate a change in the physical properties of this enzyme. It is assumed that the change is caused by a structural modification in the enzyme, arising from the substitution of one amino acid. The known properties which may be altered are the kinetics of enzyme binding to its substrate, where the enzyme has a confactor the kinetics of apoenzyme–cofactor binding and, finally, the stability of the enzyme. Examples of each of these situations will be described.

2.2.1 *Abnormal apoenzyme—substrate binding*

If a one amino acid substitution occurs in the enzyme at the active site for substrate binding it may, of course, destroy the catalytic activity completely. Alternatively, it may simply modify the site in such a way that the substrate is bound to a greater, or lesser, degree than normal. Any change in the degree of substrate binding is likely to result in decreased enzyme activity.

The most direct way of demonstrating these changes would be by making kinetic measurements on the enzyme. This has been done in a few disorders, but it is usually impossible to obtain enough reasonably pure enzyme. Citrullinaemia is one example of a disease in which it has been possible to make fairly detailed studies of the enzyme. The defect is in argininosuccinic acid synthetase, one of the enzymes involved in the urea cycle (Fig. 2.2). The disease usually

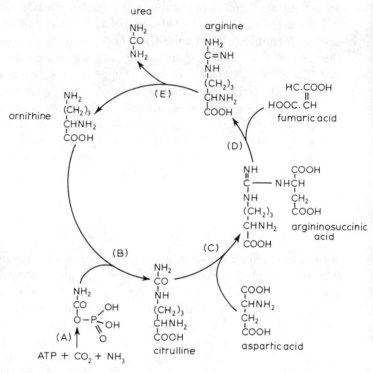

Fig. 2.2 The urea cycle. Enzymes: A, carbamyl phosphate synthetase; B, ornithine transcarbamylase; C, argininosuccinic acid synthetase; D, argininosuccinase; E, arginase.

presents with vomiting, fits and coma, the symptoms being particularly severe after a high protein meal and related to the failure to detoxify ammonia, formed by deaminating amino acids, by converting it to urea. The long-term effects of the condition include a large liver, poor growth and mental retardation.

By using tissue culture techniques sufficient material has been obtained to study the enzyme derived from patients with citrullinaemia. Fibroblast cells are grown starting from a small skin biopsy specimen. Using the enzyme isolated from these cells it has been shown that the Michaelis constant (K_m) values for citrulline and aspartic acid were increased by a factor of 40 and 500 times respectively, and in another case both K_ms were increased by 200-fold.

It may not always be necessary to carry out detailed kinetic measurements because decreases in apoenzyme–substrate affinity may be demonstrated very simply by means of a suitable competitive inhibitor. This approach is used in everyday clinical biochemistry to investigate a condition which occurs in about 1 to 2000 Caucasians, known as succinylcholine (or scoline) sensitivity. Scoline is used very widely in combination with general anaesthetics as a muscle relaxant. It is a neuromuscular blocking agent, inhibiting the action of acetylcholine at nerve endings. In the rare hypersensitive individuals the effect is too sustained and respiratory arrest may be produced by paralysis of the respiratory muscles. Initially many deaths were caused by this complication but nowadays this unfortunate outcome is usually averted by the rapid use of an artificial ventilator. Scoline is inactivated by hydrolysis to succinic acid and choline (Fig. 2.3) and

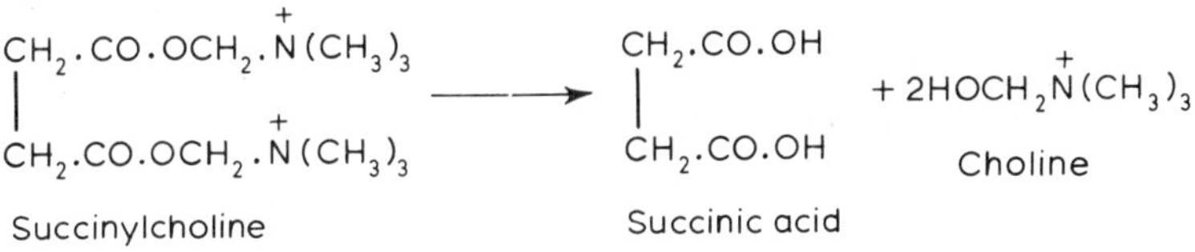

$$CH_2.CO.OCH_2.\overset{+}{N}(CH_3)_3$$
$$|$$
$$CH_2.CO.OCH_2.\overset{+}{N}(CH_3)_3$$

Succinylcholine

$$\longrightarrow$$

$$CH_2.CO.OH$$
$$|$$
$$CH_2.CO.OH$$

Succinic acid

$$+\ 2HOCH_2\overset{+}{N}(CH_3)_3$$

Choline

Fig. 2.3 Hydrolysis of succinylcholine.

this is effected by a cholinesterase present in plasma. Patients who are sensitive have only about one third of the normal plasma cholintesterase activity and it has been shown that the abnormal enzyme has an increased K_m for many choline esters as substrates. Using acetylcholine, for example, the K_m was increased six fold.

Affected individuals may be distinguished very quickly by using an

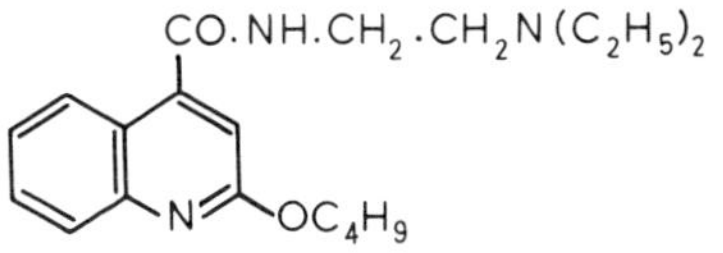

$$CO.NH.CH_2.CH_2N(C_2H_5)_2$$

$$N \diagdown OC_4H_9$$

Fig. 2.4 Dibucaine.

inhibitor in the cholinesterase assay and this is the way that the condition is usually diagnosed. The cholinesterase assay is performed with acetylcholine as substrate, with or without the addition of 10^{-5}M dibucaine (Fig. 2.4), which is a local anaesthetic, as the inhibitor. Scoline sensitive individuals have a cholinesterase which is inhibited to a lesser extent than the normal enzyme. Typical results are shown in Table 2.1

Table 2.1

Genotype of subject	Inhibition with 10^{-5}M dibucaine (%)
Normal	80
Sensitive individual, homozygous for abnormal gene	20
Heterozygous normal/abnormal gene	60

The percent inhibition, or dibucaine number as it is often called, completely characterizes the genotype of an individual with respect to scoline sensitivity.

2.2.2 *Abnormal apoenzyme–cofactor interaction*

The formation of an active enzyme is often dependent on the interaction between an apoenzyme and a specific cofactor to form a holoenzyme complex. Many inherited metabolic diseases may be explained on the basis of a structural alteration in the apoenzyme causing abnormal formation of the complex.

Indications of this problem arose initially from work on a disorder known as cystathioninuria. Although the condition was described originally in patients who had fits and were mentally retarded, it now appears that these clinical findings were not related to the biochemical abnormality and that cystathioninuria has no harmful consequences.

The defect in cystathioninuria is in the enzyme cystathioninase which is involved in the transulphuration pathway converting methionine to cystine (Fig. 2.5). Cystathioninase is a complex of four molecules of pyridoxal-5-phosphate (pyr-5-P) with one molecule of apoenzyme. Vitamin B_6 is the precursor of pyr-5-P and when it was given in very large doses to people with cystathioninuria the

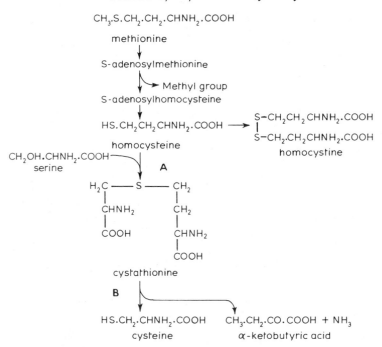

Fig. 2.5 Transulphuration pathway for the conversion of methionine to cystine. Key enzymes: A, cystathionine-β-synthase; B, γ-cystathioninase.

biochemical abnormality appeared to be corrected. The inherited condition was said to be 'vitamin responsive'. Numerous other examples of the phenomenon exist and the administration of the appropriate vitamin has become an important method of treatment.

A number of different mechanisms may explain vitamin responsiveness in the various circumstances in which it has been observed, but the possibility of abnormal apoenzyme–cofactor interaction was considered first for cystathioninuria. The hypothesis was supported by the observation that in subjects with the condition, liver cystathioninase was only 2 to 3 percent of normal in assays unsupplemented with pyr-5-P, but became about 60% of normal when very high concentrations of cofactor were included in the assay mixture. In other subjects the stimulation with the cofactor was much less and it appears that there is heterogeneity in the molecular mechanisms of the defect, even within this condition.

A more precise understanding of the problems of abnormal apoenzyme–cofactor interaction can be achieved from kinetic models in which the total enzyme reaction is represented as follows:

$$E + C \underset{k_2}{\overset{k_1}{\rightleftharpoons}} EC + S \rightleftharpoons ECS \longrightarrow EC + P$$

E = the apoenzyme, C = the cofactor, S = the substrate, P = the product, k_1 and k_2 are the rate constants for the forward and reverse reactions of the EC complex.

The simplest model assumes that the formation of the EC complex is rapid and reversible and an abnormal apoenzyme causes an increase in the k_2/k_1, ratio so that the concentration of EC is reduced in the presence of normal concentrations of cofactor. A second assumption can be made that, in spite of the abnormality of apoenzyme, the EC complex that is formed can function entirely normally in the subsequent reactions. If the conditions hold, normal enzyme activity can be restored by increasing C sufficiently to produce a normal EC concentration.

Changes in the equilibrium of the formation of the holoenzymes are reflected in the Michaelis constant (K_m) for the cofactor. Kinetic measurements have been made with methylmalonyl-CoA mutase, the defective enzyme in the disease known as methylmalonic aciduria (Fig. 2.6). This condition usually presents when an infant is very young with a profound acidosis, hypoglycaemia and hyperglycinaemia. The acidosis is due to the accumulation of propionic and

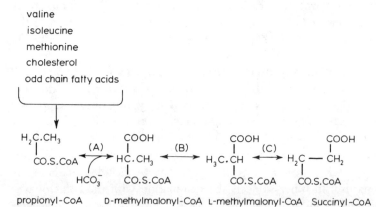

valine
isoleucine
methionine
cholesterol
odd chain fatty acids

propionyl-CoA   D-methylmalonyl-CoA   L-methylmalonyl-CoA   Succinyl-CoA

Fig. 2.6 Metabolic pathway for the conversion of propionyl-CoA to succinyl-CoA. Key enzymes: A, propionyl-CoA carboxylase; B, methylmalonyl-CoA racemase; C, methylmalonyl-CoA mutase.

methylmalonic acids and as the catabolic products of many compounds feed into this pathway the abnormality is usually very serious. The cause of the other biochemical aberrations is less well understood.

The methylmalonyl-CoA mutase requires a derivative of vitamin B_{12}, adenosyl cobalamin, as a cofactor, two molecules of cofactor combining with each molecule of apoenzyme. In some mutations of the enzyme the problem is clearly one of enzyme–cofactor interaction and enzyme prepared from the cultured skin fibroblasts of affected subjects has a K_m for adenosyl cobalamin of 50 to 500 times greater than normal.

It is quite obvious that the assumptions we have made in the model system are probably rarely applicable and the problem is far more complex. Usually the holoenzyme will not function completely normally and it would be impossible to restore the maximum velocity of the enzyme with cofactor. In some cases the complex formed with the altered apoprotein is unstable, and the protein is catabolized. Thus the concentration of the complex is reduced through its removal by an alternative route. In other cases the formation of the holoenzyme is slow and apparently irreversible and, in the extreme situation, involves covalent bond formation. For example, the holoenzyme formation of several carboxylases of interest require adenosyl biotin as cofactor in covalent linkage (for example, propionyl-CoA carboxylase, Fig. 2.6). In some of their defects abnormal formation of the complex is likely.

In spite of all the reservations about the mechanisms it seems that, in many instances, a small but very significant increase in enzyme activity may be achieved by vitamin response. Many patients with homocystinuria, a condition in which pyridoxal-5-phosphate containing cystathionine-β-synthase is defective (Fig. 2.5), respond to vitamin B_6, although the maximum stimulation of enzyme activity that can be achieved *in vitro* with high concentrations of cofactor is from an original level of 1 to 2% of normal to 3 to 4% of normal. It has been calculated that even this small improvement in activity may prevent the accumulation of methionine and homocystine by allowing normal flux of metabolites through the pathway.

2.2.3 Unstable enzymes

It is possible for a structural modification in an enzyme to affect its stability whilst leaving its functional properties intact, or almost intact. Enzyme activity may be deficient because of a net reduction in the concentration of functioning molecules.

The best demonstration of this situation exists in the disease glucose-6-phosphate dehydrogenase (Gd) deficiency. Affected individuals suffer severe haemolytic episodes following contact with certain precipitating factors. These include a wide variety of drugs, the principal groups being anti-malarials and sulphonamides; but in areas around the Mediterranean a constituent of the normal diet, the fava bean, may cause a crisis, and this has led to the condition being known as Favism in these countries. Apart from its occurrence around the Mediterranean, the disease is seen mainly in American Negroes.

The sporadic haemolytic anaemia which occurs in this condition is the result of a deficiency of Gd in the erythrocytes. The role of the enzyme in red cell metabolism is considered to be the maintenance of glutathione in its reduced form (Fig. 2.7) which is essential for the stability of the cell membrane. When there is a deficiency of Gd both the stages at which NADPH, and reduced glutathione, can be generated are affected. It appears that, in affected subjects, the erythrocyte remains stable under normal circumstances but cell

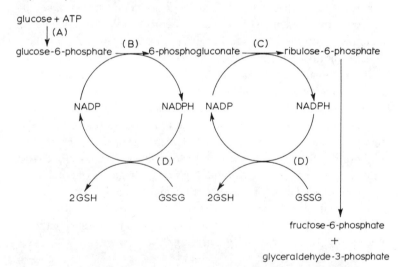

Fig. 2.7 The pentose-phosphate pathway of glucose metabolism in red cells. Key enzymes: A, hexokinase; B, glucose-6-phosphate dehydrogenase; C, 6-phosphogluconate dehydrogenase; D, glutathione reductase.

destruction ensues following contact with oxidizing substances. The level of red cell reduced glutathione is decreased by such compounds since the mechanism for regenerating it is inadequate.

The Negro and Mediterranean forms of the disease are due to different mutations of the enzyme and the latter has been studied in rather more detail. Affected individuals have about 15% of normal levels of Gd but the residual enzyme appears normal with respect to its pH optimum and all its kinetic properties. On the other hand, there is good evidence that the enzyme molecule is unstable.

It is possible to separate erythrocytes according to the time they have been circulating in the blood stream. Using this technique it was found that there was an unusually rapid decline in the concentration of Gd with ageing of the red cells of affected patients. The biological half life of the enzyme in deficient individuals was calculated to be only 13 days compared to the normal of 62 days.

It seems likely that structural instability is a frequent cause of enzyme deficiency but this may be related to defective interaction of the apoenzyme with its cofactor, or even its substrate. Enzyme stability may also be influenced by the cellular environment and it has become obvious that the red cell, which being enucleated is unable to synthesize new enzyme, and which has a very long lifespan, is particularly vulnerable to the problem.

2.3 Possible defects in the rate of enzyme synthesis

In the earlier sections of this chapter it was pointed out that investigations in the thalassaemias have indicated the possibility of defects in which either no enzyme, or a reduced amount of structurally normal enzyme, is synthesized. The mechanisms by which this type of disorder could occur, and the difficulty of demonstrating the former situation, were discussed.

A number of conditions have been postulated to be due to these rate control problems, but the claims have not been substantiated. One of the more interesting of these, which is worth considering, is a disease known as orotic aciduria. Orotic aciduria is a rare disorder in the pathway of pyrimidine nucleotide synthesis. It usually presents in the early months of life with pallor, due to a megaloblastic anaemia, and retarded growth and development. A heavy excretion of the orotic acid crystals was the clue to the biochemical basis of the disease, since it was known that the compound was an intermediate in the pyrimidine synthetic pathway.

Two findings prompted the original suggestion that orotic aciduria was a problem of gene regulation. Firstly, when the enzyme pathway was studied in red cells, it was found that two enzymes were deficient in the patients (Fig. 2.8). Secondly, investigation of the

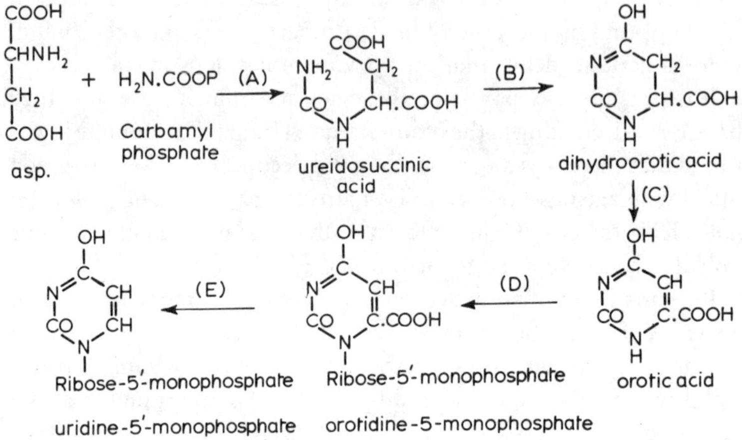

Fig. 2.8   Pathway of uridine-5'-monophophate synthesis. (Enzymes D and E are defective in orotic aciduria.) Enzymes: A, aspartate transcarbamylase; B, dihydroorotase; C, dihydroorotic acid dehydrogenase; D, orotidine-5'-monophosphate pyrophosphorylase; E, orotidine-5'-monophosphate decarboxylase.

parents also showed a fairly profound enzyme deficiency, certainly much less than the 50% of normal activity expected in obligate heterozygotes. The observation that two adjacent enzymes in the pathway were missing could be explained simply if they were both coded by genes on the same operon and abnormal regulator genes caused the transcription of both structural genes to be repressed. The low enzyme activity in the heterozygotes could be due, likewise, to the product of a single abnormal regulator gene causing transcription repression of more than 50%. However, the finding of two missing enzymes could be explained also by a large deletion which removed the genes coding for both enzymes, assuming they were situated on adjacent positions on the same chromosome.

Orotic aciduria is unique in being the only human disorder in which there appears to be an inherited defect in two enzymes, but the cause remains unclear. There is now some evidence that the two affected enzymes share a common polypeptide unit and, therefore, could both be abnormal because of a mutation in a single gene. The apparently reduced expression of the normal gene in the heterozygotes could be explained in a number of ways other than the regulator gene hypothesis, and this general problem will be discussed in the next chapter.

3

Genetic heterogeneity

3.1 Introduction

The fusion of the ideas of classical genetics and biochemistry into the subject of inherited metabolic diseases resulted in a number of basic assumptions about the nature of enzymes in various situations. These assumptions may be summarized as follows.

(1) All members of a population possessing normal activity of a particular enzyme have the same molecular species of enzyme.

(2) Patients with a clinically and biochemically distinct inborn error of metabolism are a homogeneous group of individuals with an identical variant form of the same enzyme.

(3) Qualitative and quantitative differences in the clinical expression of a specific inborn error of metabolism are due to the

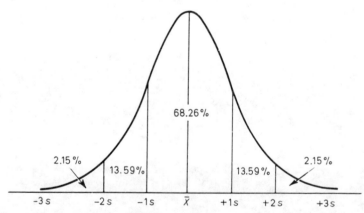

Fig. 3.1 The normal or Gaussian distribution showing the percentage of the sample occurring between certain intervals based on the standard deviation (*s*) and around the mean ($\overline{X}$).

interaction of environmental factors with the identical enzyme defect.

(4) An inherited deficiency of a particular enzyme will be present in every cell and tissue in which the enzyme is normally synthesized.

(5) There is a precise gene dosage effect determining the level of an enzyme. Thus, a heterozygote for a normal gene coding for an enzyme with 100% activity, and an abnormal gene coding for a defective enzyme with no activity, will have 50% enzyme activity.

Many people continue to study inborn errors of metabolism with these assumptions in mind but, in fact, all the ideas must be modified. In this chapter we shall consider how and why genetic variation is so much more complex, this being extremely important for an understanding of all the facts now available. It is perhaps the most interesting development in the subject in recent years.

3.2 Enzyme variation in normal individuals

3.2.1 Red cell acid phosphatase

When we measure the levels of a particular enzyme in the plasma, or cells, of a large population of healthy people the distribution of values obtained is usually 'Gaussian' or 'normal' (Fig. 3.1). Conventionally, the normal distribution is explained by variations in the rate of synthesis of a qualitatively identical enzyme in members of this population, and possibly by the presence of different amounts of inhibitors or activators modifying the enzyme activity. It has now become apparent that variation of measured enzyme levels in the normal population may also be due to genetically determined differences in the structure and properties of the polypeptide, or polypeptides, which constitute the enzyme.

Many examples of genetic heterogeneity in normal populations have been discovered, but one of the first and most carefully investigated is that of acid phosphatase in the red blood cell. The kind of acid phosphatase molecule which an individual synthesizes appears to be determined by three autosomal, allelic forms of a gene which code for three different enzymes, called types A, B and C. There are six possible phenotypes for acid phosphatase, namely homozygous A, B and C and heterozygous AB, AC and BC.

The enzymes synthesized in the different genetic types can be

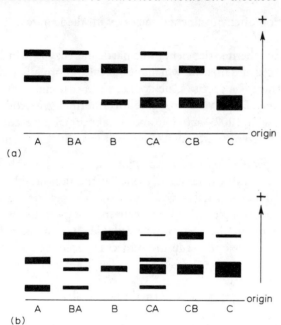

Fig. 3.2 Electrophoretic patterns of the six red cell acid phosphatase phenotypes. Starch gel electrophoresis was performed at pH 6.0 in (a) a citrate-phosphate buffer; (b) a phosphate buffer. Reproduced with permission from Harris (1980) *The Principles of Human Biochemical Genetics*, 3rd edn, Elsevier, Amsterdam.

distinguished by the patterns of migration of the polypeptides on starch gel electrophoresis which are shown in Fig. 3.2. It will be seen that each gene seems to determine two enzyme bands, but there is evidence that these are conformational isomers of the same polypeptide molecule. The important point to notice is that the heterozygote phenotypes are mixtures of the homozygous phenotypes, thus supporting the premise that the phenotypes are determined by three allelic genes. Family studies are also in agreement with the allelic gene concept. For example in 94 matings between BA heterozygotes, the possible red cell acid phosphatase phenotype of AA, AB and BB occurred in 40, 91 and 54 of the children respectively. This is close to the theoretical ratio of 1:2:1 that would be expected.

The most likely explanation for the different inherited forms of red cell acid phosphatase is that they represent single amino acid substitutions in basically the same polypeptide chain. The amino acid

Table 3.1 *Distribution and enzyme activity of red cell acid phosphatase phenotypes*

Phenotype	A	BA	B	CA	CB	C
Proportion in a normal population (%)	15.7	37.6	35.8	3.6	7.1	0.2
Mean activity*	122.4	153.9	188.3	183.8	212.3	(240.7)†
(s.d.)	(16.8)	(17.3)	(19.5)	(19.8)	(23.1)	

* μmol of *p*-nitrophenol liberated from *p*-nitrophenyl phosphate per 30 min per g Hb at 37°
† This value is extrapolated from the other data

substitution confers a charge difference on enzyme A, but the only difference between enzymes B and C is a change in the proportion of the electrophoretically slow and fast moving conformation isomers. However, it can be seen from Table 3.1 that each enzyme has a characteristic activity, so that there is increasing activity from A to C. The enzyme levels in the heterozygotes are the mean of the

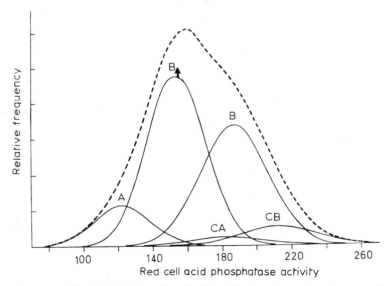

Fig. 3.3. The distribution of red cell acid phosphatase in the general population (broken line) and the contribution of the different phenotypes to the total. Reproduced with permission from Harris (1980) *The Principles of Human Biochemical Genetics*, 3rd edn, Elsevier, Amsterdam.

corresponding homozygote levels. There is some evidence that the difference in activity of the enzymes is dependent on variations in the stability of the polypeptides rather than the basic kinetic properties.

The data in Table 3.1 on the activity associated with each red cell acid phosphatase phenotype, together with the observed frequency of each in the population, can be used to show their contribution to the overall normal range (Fig. 3.3). It is clear that differences in activity in the phenotypes make a significant contribution to normal variation.

3.2.2   Other enzymes

Because of the association of glucose-6-phosphate dehydrogenase (Gd) deficiency with episodes of haemolytic anaemia, this enzyme has been studied extensively in populations in which the problem occurs. The commonest form of enzyme in all populations is designated GdB, but about 150 variants have been described which are differentiated by kinetic properties, thermostability and electrophoretic mobility. Around 96% of these variants appear to be compatible with completely normal health, although in a number of these the red cell Gd activity is very significantly reduced.

Most of the Gd variants have an extremely low incidence but three have been found much more frequently in particular populations. One of these, GdA, is present in over 20% of male Negroes and is associated with normal red cell enzyme activity. It has been established that the structural difference between the two common 'normal' alleles in Negro populations is the replacement of an asparagine in GdB by an aspartic acid in GdA. This introduces a charge difference so that the two forms of enzyme can be separated easily on electrophoresis. The other two are Gd Canton, which occurs in Southern China, and Gd Athens, from Greece. Males who have either of these variants have less than a quarter of the enzyme activity of those with the GdB phenotype.

One rare variant, Gd Hektoen, is noteworthy because people with it have four times the normal activity associated with GdB. It is known that this unusual variant is a point mutation, a histidine in GdB being replaced by a tyrosine residue in Gd Hektoen. There is evidence that the specific activity of the mutant enzyme is quite normal and its stability is not increased. It has been postulated, therefore, that the excessive Gd activity is due to an increased rate of enzyme synthesis.

It was pointed out in Chapter 1 that even enzyme variations which produce pronounced metabolic derangement may be compatible with normality and these add, therefore, to the extreme heterogeneity encountered in healthy populations. A relatively common example of this phenomenon is the amino acid disorder histidinaemia, a condition which has an interesting history.

Histidinaemia is an autosomal recessive condition caused by a deficiency of the enzyme L-histidine ammonia lyase (Fig. 3.4). Histidine accumulates in tissues and blood, and is excreted in increased concentration in urine. In addition, the unusual histidine metabolites, imidazole pyruvic acid, imidazole lactic acid and imidazole

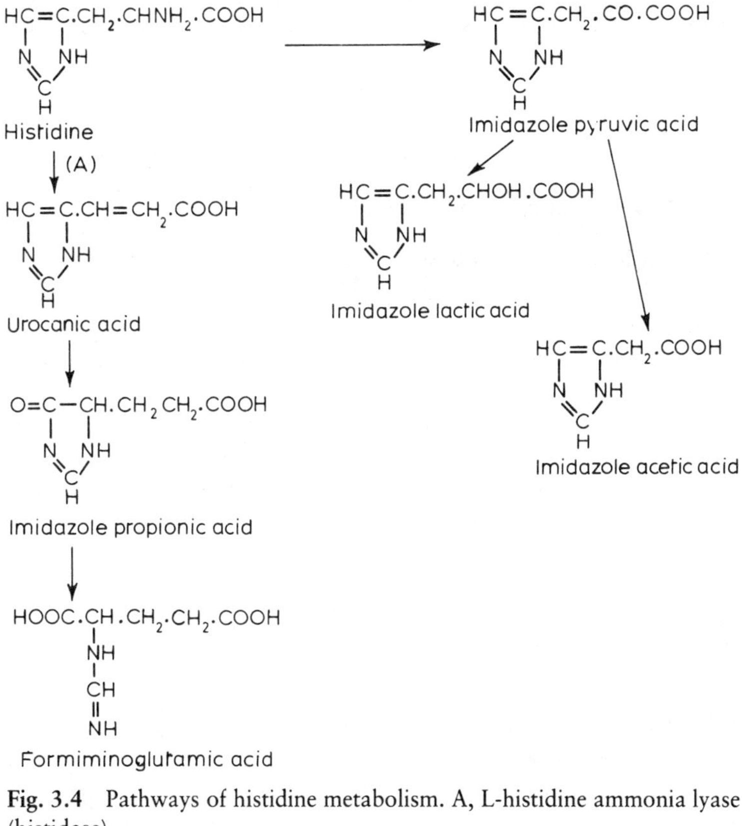

Fig. 3.4 Pathways of histidine metabolism. A, L-histidine ammonia lyase (histidase).

acetic acid are excreted. The biochemical picture is analogous to that in phenylketonuria, the disorder of phenylalanine metabolism, which does have very significant clinical effects.

Histidinaemia was first described in 1961 and the early cases were found in children with mental retardation, impaired speech, seizures, disturbed behaviour and learning problems. Doubts emerged about a causal relationship between histidinaemia and the disease findings because some siblings of the original patients were quite healthy, although they too had the biochemical disorder. In addition, some cases discovered by routine screening were normal.

Because of the questions regarding the consequences of histidinaemia several prospective studies were initiated by screening the newborn population. As a result of these studies it may be concluded that 99% of children who have histidinaemia will grow up with no abnormality relatable to their metabolic condition. Also, it cannot be proved that there is a causal relationship between histidinaemia and the central nervous system disorder in the rare cases in which these abnormalities are associated. Therefore, it seems reasonably certain that histidinaemia is a normal genetic variation.

3.3   Genetic variation in disease states

This heading can encompass both genetic variations in the biochemical phenotype and in the degree of clinical expression of a disease entity. Obviously these two factors are often directly related. The question of biochemical variation will be considered first and in greater depth.

Different biochemical phenotypes, causing essentially the same disease, may involve the same polypeptide chain and occur at the same gene locus, a phenomenon known as multiple allelism, or may involve different polypeptide chains and, therefore, multiple gene loci.

3.3.1   *Multiple allelism*

Until recently it was assumed that all patients with a particular inherited metabolic disease had a genetically homogeneous abnormality. When the levels of the affected enzyme were determined they were usually so low that they could not be confidently distinguished from zero. Therefore, there was no basis for suspecting heterogeneity.

The first indication that inherited disorders may be due to many different allelic mutations in the same polypeptide molecule came from work on abnormal haemoglobins, in particular on the variants of the haemoglobin β-chain. These variants retained the spectral characteristics of haemoglobin and could therefore be detected on electrophoresis. Molecules with different electrical charges could therefore be easily distinguished. Well over a hundred allelic mutations in the β-chain have been discovered, all but five of these varying from the normal structure by a single amino acid substitution. In exceptional cases two amino acid mutations have been present at the same time, but this is obviously a relatively rare occurrence. Calculations suggest that more than three hundred point mutations producing a charge difference in the β-chain should be possible.

There is no reason why the phenomenon of multiple allelism should not occur as frequently in enzyme abnormalities, but we have been hindered from demonstrating this because, when there is no residual catalytic activity in the molecule, there is no direct method of studying the enzyme. Some indications of the possibility of genetic heterogeneity may sometimes be found from family studies which show different patterns of metabolic abnormality in the heterozygotes for a condition. However, there is more scope to investigate the abnormal enzyme when it has significant residual activity. This is most aptly demonstrated in the case of glucose-6-phosphate dehydrogenase (see section 3.2.2). Over 150 variants of this enzyme have been described, although only seven of them cause episodic haemolytic anaemia. Another example of multiple allelism was described in Section 2.2.1 involving the enzyme arginino-succinic acid synthetase. Two forms of the disorder have been found in which the K_m for the substrates citrulline and aspartic acid are increased in quite different proportions.

A consequence of multiple allelism is that patients with an autosomal recessive disease need not be true homozygotes but are likely to be heterozygous for genes coding for two different variant forms of the affected enzyme. This situation would be unusual, however, when the parents of the child are first cousins because it is probable that both the mother and father have inherited the same abnormal gene in this case. Nor is it likely in diseases which are confined to one particular race, or population, since this usually arises through the spread of the same gene mutation due to intermarriage, or because it confers some genetic advantage. The concurrence of two variant genes in the same individual is more likely to be found in diseases which have a relatively uniform incidence in many populations, indicating the likelihood of many different mutational events.

An example of the simultaneous occurrence of two different allelic forms in a patient has been described in the deficiency of red cell pyruvate kinase which is associated with haemolytic anaemia. These studies have shown that patients are usually heterozygous for one gene which codes for an enzyme with negligible activity, and one which leads to the synthesis of an enzyme with measurable activity. The latter may be qualitatively differentiated from normal by its kinetic properties, or its electrophoretic mobility. The findings can often be reinforced by similar studies in the mother and father of the patient.

Another rather interesting example of multiple allelism in the same patient involved children with a variant, or atypical, form of phenylketonuria (PKU). PKU is one of the best known, and well studied, inborn errors of metabolism and is a disorder in the catabolism of the amino acid phenylalanine. It was first described in 1934 by a Norwegian doctor named Følling. There is a defect in the apoenzyme of phenylalanine-4-hydroxylase, which is involved in the hydroxylation of phenylalanine in the para position to form tyrosine (Fig. 3.5). It appears that in the typical form of PKU there is virtually no ability to metabolize phenylalanine, which leads to a big increase in concentration of the amino acid in body fluids and the production, and excretion, of unusual metabolites phenyl pyruvic, lactic and acetic acids. The most disturbing aspect of PKU is the almost invariable development of very severe mental handicap. Other features include vomiting, lethargy, fits, eczema and fair skin and hair. About thirty years ago it was shown that all the disease symptoms could be prevented by early treatment with a special diet, restricted in its phenylalanine content.

More recently newborn screening was introduced for PKU, so that treatment was most effective by starting it early. Screening, by measuring blood phenylalanine, has resulted in the discovery of many children with variant, or atypical, forms of PKU, in which the accumulation of phenylalanine was less pronounced than in the typical, or 'classical', form of the disease. It is probable that, like pyruvate kinase deficiency, children with the variant forms of PKU are heterozygous for a classical PKU gene, coding for an apoenzyme with negligible function, and a mutant gene which allows the

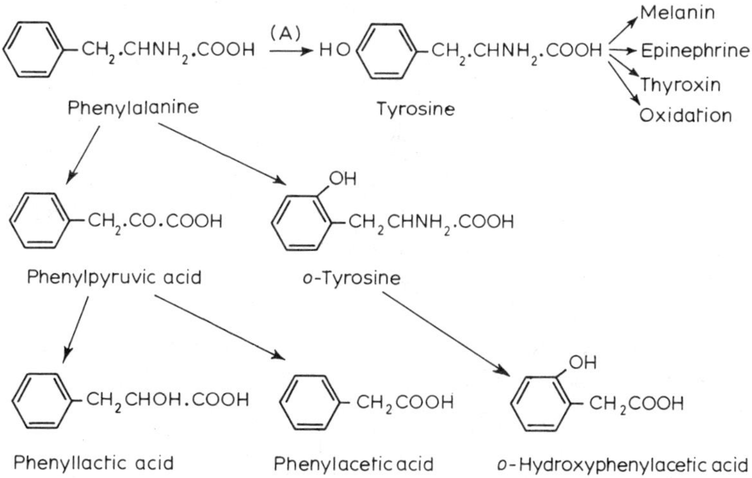

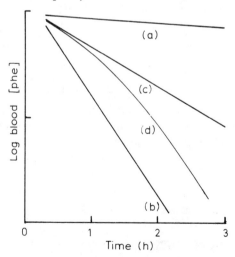

Fig. 3.5 Pathways of phenylalanine metabolism. A, phenylalanine hydroxylase.

synthesis of an apoenzyme having significant activity. Thus there is some capacity to metabolize phenylalanine.

A number of atypical PKU families have been studied by following decay curves of blood phenylalanine after an intravenous infusion of

Fig. 3.6 The rate of fall of blood phenylalanine following an intravenous infusion of the amino acid in: (a) phenylketonuric subjects; (b) normal subjects; (c) heterozygotes for phenylketonuria; (d) parents of children with 'atypical' phenylketonuria.

this amino acid. In normal subjects the log of phenylalanine concentration fell rapidly and linearly over a period of three to four hours back to the original level (Fig. 3.6). In classical PKU patients there was virtually no drop in blood phenylalanine over this period, reflecting the absence of hydroxylase activity. Parents of these patients, who are obligate heterozygotes for the normal and the classical PKU genes had a decay rate which was midway between the patient's and that found in normal subjects signifying that they had approximately 50% hydroxylase activity.

In two families with an atypical PKU child, one parent of each had the usual blood phenylalanine decay characteristics of the heterozygote, but the other had an unusual biphasic curve which had the usual heterozygote slope initially and finally approached the decay slope of the normal person (Fig. 3.6). The probable explanation for this finding is that the 'unusual' parent had one gene which coded for a variant of phenylalanine hydroxylase which was inhibited by high concentrations of its substrate. The children who were heterozygous for the classical PKU gene, contributing an enzyme with negligible activity, and the unusual gene, producing the enzyme which is inhibited by its substrate, may have a severe impairment of phenylalanine metabolism when faced with a heavy load of amino acids, but may be able to meet more normal demands.

3.3.2 *Multiple loci*

There are two ways in which a metabolic disorder may be determined by different, non-allelic, gene loci. In the first of these the disease is caused by different abnormal genes affecting the same enzyme. This can happen when the enzyme is formed by the post-translational association of more than one kind of polypeptide chain, each being coded for by an independant gene locus.

In the second situation similar biochemical and clinical consequences arise from mutations affecting different enzymes, or transport systems, which are, however, involved closely in the same metabolic pathway.

The first of these phenomena can be illustrated by reference to the enzyme N-acetylhexosaminidase (hexosaminidase, or Hex) deficiencies of which cause Tay Sachs and Sandhoff diseases. In these diseases there is a similar rapid neurological degeneration which becomes evident in the early months of life and in both of them there is an accumulation in the brain of a specific glycosphingolipid, called GM_2 ganglioside (Fig. 3.7). The term GM_2 gangliosidosis is often used to describe the diseases.

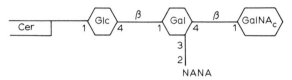

Fig. 3.7 Structure of GM_2 ganglioside, Cer, ceramide (*N*-acylsphingosine); Glc, glucose; Gal, galactose; GalNAc, *N*-acetylgalactosamine; NANA, *N*-acetylneuraminic acid.

Studies of hexosaminidase have revealed that there are two isoenzyme forms, called Hex A and B. The isoenzymes may be separated by a variety of techniques, but they can also be easily estimated individually because Hex A activity is destroyed by heating it at 50° for 1 h, whereas Hex B is relatively heat stable. Hex A is the important isoenzyme for degrading GM_2 ganglioside. Hex A will split off the terminal *N*-acetyl galactosamine from GM_2 ganglioside, whereas Hex B will only hydrolyze the terminal residue following the removal of the branched *N*-acetyl neuraminic acid (Fig. 3.7).

The biochemical difference between Tay Sachs and Sandhoff diseases was apparent when Hex A and Hex B were estimated separately. Whereas both diseases have a deficiency of Hex A, Hex B activity is present in Tay Sachs but absent in Sandhoff disease. The explanation for the biochemical heterogeneity was found by investigating the molecular structures of Hex A and B. This showed that Hex A was a polymer of two kinds of polypeptide chain (α and β) and its probable formula was $\alpha\beta_2$. Hex B was a tetramer of β chains only (β_4).

Genetic heterogeneity occurs in GM_2 gangliosidosis because the important deficiency of Hex A isomer can be due to a mutational abnormality in α-chain synthesis, as in Tay Sachs disease, or in β-chain synthesis, when Hex B will also be deficient, as in Sandhoff disease. It is now known that the gene locus for α-chains is on chromosome 15, and for β-chains is on chromosome 5. Thus the same clinical and biochemical phenotype is produced by mutations on two different chromosomes.

The GM_2 gangliosides also provide an example of the other kind of genetic heterogeneity due to multiple loci, that is where a defect in two completely different functional proteins, or enzymes, produces the same biochemical phenotype. There is only one type of GM_2 gangliosidosis in which the hexosaminidases are absolutely normal when they are measured, as is usually the practice, using a synthetic substrate. It appears that in order to hydrolyze the natural substrate, GM_2 ganglioside, Hex A requires a protein activator and it is this which is defective in the variant form of the disease. The activator protein has been isolated from human kidneys and contains two polypeptides with molecular weights of 25 000 and 60 000 daltons. The smallest of these polypeptides was absent in the kidney of a patient with the activator deficiency type of GM_2 gangliosidosis.

A more complex and well investigated example of heterogeneity in the genetic determination of the cause of a biochemical disorder is afforded by methylmalonic aciduria, (Section 2.2.2. and Fig. 2.6). The enzyme which metabolizes methylmalonic acid is methyl malonic acid mutase (mutase), the holoenzyme of which is composed of two identical, 77 500 dalton, subunits and two molecules of a cofactor, adenosyl cobalamin (AdoCbl), which is derived from vitamin B_{12}. Numerous allelic mutants of the apoenzyme appear to exist which have been broadly classified into two classes depending on whether they have zero, or measurable, catalytic potential. The enzyme forms have been differentiated further with the aid of an antibody to normal mutase. It was found that some zero activity mutants had no cross reactivity with the antibody, whereas others had some, though always subnormal, cross reactivity. All the mutants with measurable levels of mutase reacted with the antibody and they all had an altered interaction between apoenzyme and cofactor as shown by an increased K_m for AdoCbl, ranging from 50 to 5000 times normal.

It is not possible to have non-allelic mutants of the mutase apoenzyme because it is composed of two identical polypeptide subunits, but they do arise in a number of forms of methylmalonic aciduria due essentially to a deficiency of enzyme cofactor, AdoCbl. Deficiencies of AdoCbl are known to occur for two principal reasons:

(1) Because of defects in the absorption of the vitamin form, hydroxy cobalamin (OH-Cbl) in the ileum.

(2) Because of defects in the intracellular processing of OH-Cbl to AdoCbl.

The absorption of vitamin B_{12} requires the production of intrinsic factor by the stomach and specific cell membrane receptors in the ileum. Two inherited defects in intrinsic factor production have been described and one disorder of the membrane receptors. Patients with these conditions have a generalized abnormality in all processes requiring B_{12}, including the metabolism of methylmalonic acid, and their problems may be overcome by giving them OH-Cbl parenterally.

The intracellular conversion of OH-Cbl to AdoCbl, and the other important vitamin B_{12} coenzyme form methyl cobalamin (MeCbl), is illustrated in Fig. 3.8. It should be emphasized that there remains considerable uncertainty about many details of this scheme, and intramitochondrial reduction and adenosylation are the best established steps.

The transport and uptake of OH-Cbl is dependent on two proteins known as transcobalamins (TC). TCII-OH-Cbl complex is particularly involved in uptake, first being attached to a cell membrane receptor and then absorbed by endocytosis. Once within the cell the

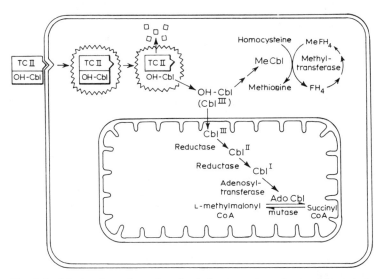

Fig. 3.8 Mechanism of uptake of cobalamin and synthesis of the cobalamin coenzymes. TCII, transcobalamin II; OH-Cbl, hydroxycobalamin; MeCbl, methyl cobalamin; MeFH$_4$, methyl tetrahydrofolate; FH$_4$ tetrahydrofolate; Cbl^{III}, Cbl^{II}, Cbl^{I}, cobalamins with valencies of 3, 2 and 1; AdoCbl, adenosyl cobalamin. Reproduced with permission from Rosenberg (1980) in *Inborn Errors of Metabolism in Humans* (eds F. Cockburn and R. Gitzelman), MTP Press, Lancaster, p. 46.

OH-Cbl is released from the complex and into the cytosol by lysosomal hydrolases. Although there are obviously many possibilities for inherited defects in these steps, none have been discovered.

Four non-allelic mutant defects have been described which affect the processing of cytosolic OH-Cbl to AdoCbl, causing methylmalonic aciduria. These have been designated A, B, C and D. In C and D there is apparently a deficiency of AdoCbl and MeCbl and it is assumed that the defects occur at points in the cytosolic pathway common to the synthesis of both the cofactors. Mutants A and B cause methylmalonic aciduria specifically, and presumably only the mitochondrial production of AdoCbl is affected. There is evidence that mutant A is a defect in one of the reductases which catalyses the successive change in the cobalt atom from valency $3+$ to $1+$, prior to the adenosylation, and that mutant B is due to a deficiency of the adenosyl transferase.

Thus the biochemical and clinical phenotype of methylmalonic aciduria can be caused by probable numerous allelic mutations in the mutase apoenzyme, but also by seven documented non-allelic mutations. Three of these mutations prevent the absorption of the vitamin precursor of the enzyme cofactor and four are defects in the conversion of the precursor to the cofactor.

3.4   Heterogeneity in the expression of an enzyme defect in different cell types

In the introduction to this chapter it was stated that, according to classical ideas, it was expected that a person with a genetic defect in a specific enzyme would have the metabolic abnormality in every cell, or tissue, in which the enzyme was normally present. In fact, the enzyme defect may be expressed in only one or two cell types. This is important practically because a defect might be more serious if it occurred throughout the body. In the extreme situation a disorder may be completely benign, because the lack of the enzyme is of no consequence in a particular type of cell, but may be lethal if the defect is expressed in another type in which the enzyme is essential. There are at least three ways in which this apparent anomaly can arise.

3.4.1   Mutiple enzymes

In some instances that enzyme which catalyses the identical

metabolic reaction is determined by a completely separate gene locus in different cell types. A good example of this is phosphorylase which catalyses the first reaction in the glycogenolytic pathway to produce glucose-1-phosphate.

A lack of phosphorylase causes an accumulation of glycogen, or glycogen storage, in the tissues involved. There are essentially two well differentiated kinds of glycogen storage depending whether the phosphorylase deficiency occurs in liver, or muscle.

Liver and muscle phosphorylase deficiency have different metabolic and physical consequences. The importance of liver glycogen is as a store of glucose which can later be mobilized to maintain the blood glucose level. A patient who lacks phosphorylase is less able to maintain the blood glucose within normal limits and develops neurological symptoms on fasting due to a shortage of energy supply to the brain. Muscle glycogen, on the other hand, provides a ready internal source of glucose when it is required rapidly during vigorous muscular activity. Patients with muscle phosphorylase deficiency are able to sustain low levels of physical activity, presumably through glucose uptake from blood, but their muscles go into painful spasms when attempting vigorous exercise. Therefore, there are two quite distinct metabolic and clinical entities depending on whether the gene locus for muscle, or liver phosphorylase is abnormal.

3.4.2 *Multilocus enzymes*

A rather similar, but more complex, situation can occur when an enzyme is a polymer of several independently inherited polypeptide units. Various combinations of subunits may form the active enzyme, as described for the hexosaminidases (section 3.3.2), but certain polymeric forms often predominate in particular forms of cell. A genetic mutation in one of the subunits may affect mainly one enzyme polymer and cause a deficient activity in only the cells which normally contain this molecular form. The enzyme phosphofructokinase (PFK) illustrates this well.

PFK is a key enzyme in the glycolytic pathway of carbohydrate metabolism, catalysing the conversion of fructose-1-phosphate to fructose-1, 6-diphosphate. Disorders of PFK have been described in muscle and erythrocytes. The muscle disease is almost identical to those of muscle phosphorylase deficiency (described in Section 3.4.1). PFK deficiency in red cells is one of many enzyme disorders which cause an haemolytic anaemia.

PFK usually exists as a tetramer and this may be composed of three kinds of subunit which have been described in humans: namely M, muscle type; L, liver type; and F, found in fibroblasts, platelets, brain, lymphocytes and kidney. Muscle contains only M subunits and its enzyme will have the structure M_4. On the other hand, erythrocytes PFK is a mixture of five isoenzymes whose structures are those expected from a random association of approximately equal amounts of M and L units – M_4, M_3L, M_2L_2, ML_3, L_4. These five isomers can be separated by chromatographic techniques.

Two kinds of PFK deficiency have been described. The most common affects both muscle and red cells which have enzyme levels of zero and about 50% of normal respectively. This form can be explained by a genetic defect in the M subunit and is supported by finding only the L_4 isoenzyme in the abnormal erythrocytes. The rarer form affects only erythrocytes and, again, they have about half normal activity. The most probable reason for this disorder is a defect in the L subunit.

3.4.3   Unstable enzymes

A defect in an enzyme which primarily affects its stability can be manifest to varying degrees in different cell types, or tissues. This may be because some cell environments are particularly good, or bad, in maintaining the activity of the altered enzyme; but, also, there is likely to be a greater net enzyme deficiency in cells with a long life span, and lower rates of protein turnover. As mentioned in Chapter 2, the erythrocyte appears most vulnerable because of its 120 day life and its inability to synthesize protein.

The Negro variant of erythrocyte Gd deficiency has been described (Section 2.2.3) in which the defect causes a rapid breakdown of the enzymes. The same patients have a minimal reduction in leucocyte Gd activity, presumably because the cells are nucleated and continue enzyme synthesis. However, since Gd is very important in red cell metabolism the defect is of clinical significance.

Some red cell enzyme deficiencies occur, however, which are of no apparent consequence. One such affects the enzyme uridine diphosphate galactose-4-epimerase (epimerase), an enzyme which plays a key role in two possible pathways of galactose metabolism (Fig. 3.9). Many people have been found who have the erythrocyte epimerase

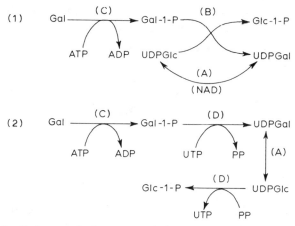

Fig. 3.9 Pathways of galactose metabolism. Two possible pathways for the metabolism of galactose to glucose-1-phosphate both involving the enzyme A, uridine diphosphate galactose-4-epimerase; B is transferase, C is galactokinase, D is pyrophosphorylase. Pathway (1) is the most well established.

deficiency but no ill effects can be related to it. The available evidence suggests that the abnormal apoenzyme in the deficient subjects has a reduced affinity for NAD (the cofactor), and this also imparts instability to the molecule. This particularly affects the erythrocyte epimerase, but it is of no real importance in the function of this cell. A number of other cell types, including those of liver, which is the principal site of galactose metabolism in the body, had virtually normal epimerase activity. A second epimerase variant has now been described in which there is a complete enzyme deficiency in all sources examined, including the liver. As might be expected, the child had an impaired capacity to metabolize galactose and had a very acute illness which could be explained by the biochemical defect.

3.5 Variable enzyme expression in heterozygotes

3.5.1 Gene dosage

In the majority of metabolic disorders it has been found that the level of enzyme activity in heterozygotes, who possess one abnormal and one normal gene, lies very close to the mid-point between the activity found in homozygous normals and homozygous abnormals, who have two normal and two abnormal genes respectively. The most frequent situation is one in which the homozygous abnormal individual has negligible enzyme activity, in which case the heterozygote has approximately 50% of the homozygous normal level. It appears as if each gene exerts its effect on the control of enzyme synthesis independently and equal quantities of normal and abnormal enzyme are made. Each gene makes a proportionate contribution to the level of enzyme activity and a simple 'gene dosage' relationship is said to hold.

3.5.2   Variations from a simple gene dosage relationship

A number of disorders have been described in which the simple gene dosage relationship does not hold. In most of these the enzyme level in the heterozygote is much lower than expected. Two conditions in which this may occur have already been described: namely, homocystinuria, or cystathionine synthase deficiency (Section 2.2.2), and histidinaemia (Section 3.2.2). Not all families exhibiting an apparently identical enzyme defect show the same gene dosage relationship. The characteristic enzyme level in heterozygotes may vary in different families. As described above, in one family with histidinaemia heterozygotes had L-histidine ammonia lyase levels of only a quarter of those in homozygous normal individuals. In other families the more usual 50% of normal activity has been found. It is presumed that these variable gene dosage effects may be explained by different enzyme forms in the families.

In some disorders the enzyme level in heterozygotes is much higher than it would be assuming simple gene dosage, for example in catalase deficiency. This condition, in which the enzyme responsible for destroying hydrogen peroxide is defective, is usually associated with ulceration of the mucosa of the nose and mouth, often developing into serious oral gangrene. Acatalasia is found mainly in Switzerland and Japan and it is apparent that different mutations occur in the two countries. The two mutations display, amongst other things, different gene dosage relationships. In the Japanese form heterozygotes have the expected 50% activity of the simple gene dosage relationship; whereas in the Swiss variant heterozygote activity is from 60 to 80% of normal.

3.5.3 *Reasons why simple gene dosage relationships do not hold*

There is no experimental evidence to explain why heterozygotes in some conditions have more, or less, enzyme activity than expected from simple gene dosage. However, it is possible to suggest a number of hypothetical mechanisms by which the phenomenon could occur.

The first possibility which should be considered is that it is an artefact introduced by the assay procedure. Suppose, for example, the abnormal enzyme is inhibited by its substrate and the substrate – velocity relationships for normal and abnormal enzymes are as shown in Fig. 3.10. If the assay is carried out at a substrate concentration of (a) the abnormal homozygote will have no enzyme activity. However, in the heterozygote the normal enzyme may deplete the substrate concentration to a point (b) at which the abnormal enzyme has some activity. In this situation, the heterozygote would have more than 50% of the normal enzyme level. Clearly assay conditions must be examined very carefully to eliminate this type of problem.

The second possibility, which has been mentioned previously (Section 2.3), is that a departure from the simple gene dosage effect could occur in disorders which are due to abnormalities in a regulator gene. In the heterozygote the product of only one mutant regulator gene could conceivably suppress the overall rate of

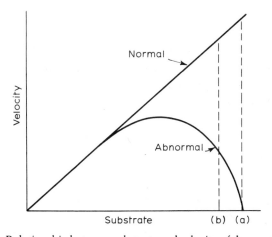

Fig. 3.10 Relationship between substrate and velocity of the reaction in the assay of an enzyme and its abnormal variant such that an artefactual gene-dosage relationship may be inferred.

transcription of the two structural genes for an enzyme by more, or less, than 50%.

The final explanation concerns those enzymes which are polymers of several polypeptide units. The simplest situation is where the enzyme is composed of two identical polypeptides A which associate freely after their synthesis. The homozygous normal can form only A subunits which associate to form the active enzyme molecule A_2, whereas the individual who is homozygous for the abnormal gene produces a variant subunit A^* which can form a dimer A^*_2, though this is inactive. The heterozygote makes both A and A^* polypeptides which will associate to form three types of polymer A_2, A^*_2 and AA^* in the ratio 1:1:2 respectively. It is quite likely that, for some reason, all molecules containing A^* are inactive. It may be that an abnormal conformation obscures the active site of the enzyme, or makes the molecule extremely unstable. In this case, the heterozygote will have only one in four active enzyme molecules and 25% of normal enzyme activity. Many enzymes are polymers of identical, or non-identical subunits and variations of this simple model are feasible explanations of many of the departures from the simple gene dosage relationship.

3.5.4 *The biochemical and clinical expression of the abnormal gene in heterozygotes*

The secondary biochemical and clinical consequences of possessing only one normal gene are not necessarily related directly to the proportion of normal enzyme synthesized. It depends, also, on how much enzyme is actually necessary to maintain normal biochemical homeostasis and clinical health. For some enzymes the normal activity may be only just adequate to meet the metabolic demands placed upon it; more often an enzyme is present in vast excess and a few per cent of normal enzyme activity is all that is required to maintain normal metabolism and health.

Slight aberrations in metabolism can often be detected in heterozygotes, however, although these have no harmful effect. For example, in phenylketonuria (Section 3.3.1) the mean level of plasma phenylalanine, or the plasma ratio of phenylalanine to tyrosine, is significantly higher in a group of heterozygotes compared to the range for the normal population. Similar situations exist in many disorders which are nevertheless regarded as having a recessive mode of inheritance from the point of view of clinical expression.

It is unusual for the heterozygote to have marked biochemical and disease characteristics and the number of metabolic disorders with dominant inheritance are few. When they do occur it is very rare to encounter the homozygous state, possibly because of the lower incidence than the heterozygous form but, more likely, because it is so severe that it results in early intrauterine death.

The effect of gene dosage on clinical expression is seen rather well in the X-linked disorder, ornithine transcarbamylase (OTC) deficiency. OTC is the second enzyme in the urea cycle (Fig. 2.2.) and its deficiency causes symptoms of vomiting, lethargy, fits and coma, related to the failure to remove ammonia from the body. There is a marked difference between males and females with the disease. In males the neurological damage is so severe that death frequently ensues in the first few days of life. The symptoms are variable but generally less serious in females, and they can usually be controlled by a moderate reduction in protein intake. There is rarely permanent neurological damage.

The sex difference in severity is related to the gene dose in males and females and a consequent difference in the degree of OTC deficiency. As the enzyme is determined by a gene on the X-chromosome affected males have no normal gene and can synthesize only abnormal enzyme. They have a severe enzyme deficiency. Affected females, on the other hand, are invariably heterozygous carriers and have, potentially, one normal and one abnormal gene per cell. Therefore, on the whole, affected females will have more active enzyme than affected males.

The situation in females is rather more complex than this because of the Lyon hypothesis (Section 1.3). Usually only the genes on one of the female X chromosomes is active in each cell. In the female patient with OTC deficiency either the normal or abnormal gene may be active and different patients will have a varying proportion of cells with active normal genes. Thus, the clinical presentation varies quite considerably in females, although generally less severe than in males.

3.6 Variations in clinical expression

A final intriguing aspect of the inherited metabolic disorders is the wide variation in the presentation of the disease in an apparently biochemically homogeneous group of patients. Two examples may illustrate this point:

(1) In phenylketonuria (Section 3.3.1) the most disturbing feature is mental retardation. Although the majority of untreated patients have an IQ below 50, the range of intelligence covers the whole spectrum and a very small proportion are intellectually normal.

(2) In the severest form of homocystinuria (Section 2.2.1) there are serious eye and skeletal abnormalities, severe mental retardation and life theatening episodes of thrombosis. On the other hand, many patients appear normal apart from the eye and minor skeletal problems.

It is possible to postulate many factors which could explain this clinical variation, including the interaction of the rest of the patient's metabolic make-up with the specific biochemical defect and an influence of environmental factors. Interesting though these possibilities are, there is little positive evidence on their contribution to the problem. However, there are three more tangible factors which require a brief consideration. They are biochemical heterogeneity, diet and infections.

3.6.1   Biochemical heterogeneity affecting clinical expression

It is clear that marked degrees of biochemical heterogeneity will be associated with clinical variation. However, most diseases occur in patients with apparently negligible enzyme activity and it is assumed that they represent a biochemically homogeneous group. Unfortunately most assays are incapable of distinguishing enzyme levels of say 5% of normal, from zero. Yet it has been proposed that an increase in enzyme activity from 1 or 2% to 3 or 4% of normal is enough to correct the secondary metabolic abnormalities of, and to treat, homocystinuria. This suggests that very minor degrees of enzyme heterogeneity, which may not be detectable by most assay techniques, could explain some observed clinical variations.

3.6.2   Diet

The secondary biochemical changes and pathological consequences of many inherited metabolic disorders arise through the metabolism of components of a normal diet. A very large number of defects occur in the metabolic pathways of amino acids, lipids and the carbohydrates, galactose and fructose. The extent of the metabolic abnormality in these defects will probably vary depending on the amount of protein, lipid, or offending carbohydrate, in the diet, and this may then influence the clinical severity in the patient. In some cases, disorders which usually present in an acute and life threatening form are not manifest for many years because of an unusual dietary situation.

Attempts to correlate the degree of metabolic abnormality with clinical abnormality have not been very successful. In phenylketonuria, for example, the level of blood phenylalanine, or other abnormal urine metabolites, has been compared with IQ. It has to be remembered, however, that the intellectual impairment relates to the extent of the metabolic abnormality in the past. In PKU, the brain is most vulnerable to damage in the first few months of life and becomes successively more able to withstand the metabolic insult as time ensues.

3.6.3 Infection

Many patients with an inherited metabolic defect present for the first time, or have recurrent attacks, when they have an infection. An infection may stress the patient's metabolism in many ways, but one specific factor affects a large number of defects. This is the tremendous tissue catabolism which is usually associated with infectious illness. In particular, there is a big increase in protein catabolism which may precipitate a crisis in disorders of amino acid metabolism.

4

Secondary
biochemical consequences
and pathogenic mechanisms
in the inherited
metabolic diseases

4.1 Introduction

In this chapter some of the wider effects of an alteration in the primary structure of a protein will be examined, and the ways in which these may explain the overt signs of the disease process associated with particular mutations. It should be admitted, at the onset, that there are very few disorders in which there is a complete understanding of the pathogenic mechanisms.

There are, however, good reasons for the poor progress in this area. Firstly, there are inherent limitations to experimental studies in the living human. Unfortunately, tissues obtained at post-mortem are rarely able to contribute useful information. Often a tissue looks surprisingly normal by all microscopic techniques or, alternatively, may be completely distorted by years of metabolic insult so that the initial pathological process is obscured. Post-mortem tissues are not good for biochemical studies unless they are obtained extremely rapidly after death. Secondly, very few true animal models of human metabolic diseases exist, and setting up an accurate experimental model is almost impossible. Finally, although work with an *in vitro* system may produce many possible explanations for a disease process, it is difficult to know whether they really happen *in vivo*.

The state of knowledge regarding secondary consequences of the inherited protein defects and specific pathogenic mechanisms will be considered under three headings. First, a rather specialized effect in which a change in primary structure leads to failure to attach identity markers, and a consequent abnormality in distribution of the protein. Second, the enzyme defects discussed in Chapter 2 result in well-defined abnormalities in cellular metabolism which may be the direct cause of pathological changes. Third, presumed similar effects in proteins involved in membrane transport may lead to the development of disease processes.

4.2 Distribution defects

4.2.1 Alpha$_1$-antitrypsin deficiency

A significant portion of cases of emphysema, or destructive lung diseases, and liver cirrhosis, occurring in adults, and hepatitis in newborn infants, are associated with a genetically determined deficiency of plasma alpha$_1$-antitrypsin. About 95% of the normal population is homozygous for an alpha$_1$-antitrypsin, or protease inhibitor, type M. Their genotype is abbreviated as PiMM. The most important deficiency allele is designated Z, and the diseases described occur mainly in homozygous, PiZZ, individuals. The Pi type may be distinguished easily by the differing electrophoretic mobilities of the corresponding proteins.

Originally it seemed likely that alpha$_1$-antitrypsin deficiency could be explained by a reduced rate of synthesis, or by the production of a structurally abnormal protein which was a less efficient protease inhibitor. The site of alpha$_1$-antitrypsin synthesis is the rough endoplasmic reticulum of the liver cell, whence the protein moves to the Golgi apparatus for secretion by vesicles formed within the Golgi, and transported in the plasma to sites within the body. When it was discovered that those with the PiZZ genotype alpha$_1$-antitrypsin accumulated in cytoplasmic inclusions in the liver cell, it became apparent that there was a problem of movement within, or secretion from, the liver. In other words, it was a distribution defect.

Alpha$_1$-antitrypsin is composed of a single polypeptide chain of about 200 amino acids, with three or four oligosaccharide side-chains attached to asparagine residues. The total molecular weight is about 52 000 dalton and 10 to 15% of this is carbohydrate. The abnormal glycoprotein in PiZZ individuals was found to contain 30% less carbohydrate than normal, and this was thought originally to be the primary defect. Sequencing of the polypeptide chains has now revealed an amino acid change in the protein product found in PiZZ individuals, a lysine at the 53rd position from the C-terminal end replacing a glutamic acid in normal alpha$_1$-antitrypsin. It is presumed that this point mutation leads to a conformational change in the protein, which prevents the post-translational attachment of one of the oligosaccharide side-chains.

It is probable that the absence of an oligosaccharide side-chain may directly explain the distribution defect of the abnormal alpha$_1$-antitrypsin. It is well established that carbohydrate attachments act as identity markers, determining the transport of glycoprotein between the organelles, and secretion from the cell. Thus, at some point, the transport of synthesized abnormal alpha$_1$-antitrypsin into the circulation is interrupted.

The liver disease which may occur in PiZZ individuals is believed to be related to the accumulation of glycoprotein in cytoplasmic inclusions. Consistent with this hypothesis is the observation of other forms of alpha$_1$-antitrypsin deficiency, in which the protein does not accumulate in the liver and that are not associated with hepatic disease. The precise links between the inclusions of alpha$_1$-antitrypsin and liver damage have not been elucidated.

Much more may be said about the pathogenesis of the lung disease in the PiZZ patient. The distribution defect causes an actual deficiency of alpha$_1$-antitrypsin in the lung. However, alpha$_1$-antitrypsin is a misnomer, which hides the protein's significance in this organ. It has, in fact, a very broad range of inhibitory activity against proteases, and its affinity for trypsin is much less than for several other enzymes; one of particular importance, with respect to the present discussion, is elastase. Elastase hydrolyzes elastin which is a key constituent of the connective tissue of the lung alveolus, giving it elastic properties. The lung of the PiZZ individual, deficient in protease inhibitor, is particularly vulnerable to attack by elastase. The source of the damaging elastase is neutrophils which, under certain circumstances, may infiltrate the lung from the circulation.

The elastase hypothesis for the pathogenesis of destructive lung disease is supported by considerable experimental evidence, including the observation that animals which have elastase instilled into their lungs develop a lung lesion like emphysema. A role of smoking in predisposing the PiZZ individual to more severe emphysema is also explained, as it has been found to increase neutrophil infiltration into the lungs.

4.2.4 I-cell disease

I-cell disease is one of a large number of inherited conditions known collectively as lysosomal storage diseases. These diseases are due typically to the deficiency of one of the hydrolases which are found within lysosomes, and which have the function of 'digesting' and removing a wide range of macromolecules from the cell. The two principal kinds of defects are those involving the enzymes which degrade the mucopolysaccharides, dermatan sulphate, heparan sulphate and keratan sulphate (Fig. 4.1), which are important components of connective tissues, and the sphingolipids (see, for example, Fig. 3.7); but also simple lipases and proteases may be affected. The deficiency of a lysosomal enzyme causes an intracellular accumulation of a particular macromolecule, and this disrupts the function of the tissues concerned. A storage disease frequently has very widespread, and severe, clinical consequences.

The symptoms of I-cell disease are very similar to those of the better known mucopolysaccharide disorder, Hurler disease (see Fig. 4.1), but the former condition presents much earlier in life. Hurler disease has been referred to commonly as gargoylism, because of the characteristic, coarse featured, appearance. Both diseases have other much more serious symptoms, including growth retardation, corneal opacities, skeletal abnormalities, large liver and spleen, and retarded mental development. Death usually occurs in the first, or second, decade.

It became apparent that I-cell disease was fundamentally different to Hurler disease because cultured skin fibroblasts from I-cell patients were shown to contain certain very remarkable dense inclusions, on phase contrast microscopy. These cellular inclusions gave the disease its name. Furthermore, it was found to be an unusual example of a storage disease because, not one, but many lysosomal enzymes were deficient. The affected enzymes were of many different classes, and included glycosidases, sulphatases and cathepsins. It would be expected that several types of macromolecules would accumulate.

The basis of the multiple hydrolase deficiency in I-cell disease was indicated when it was found that patients had abnormally high

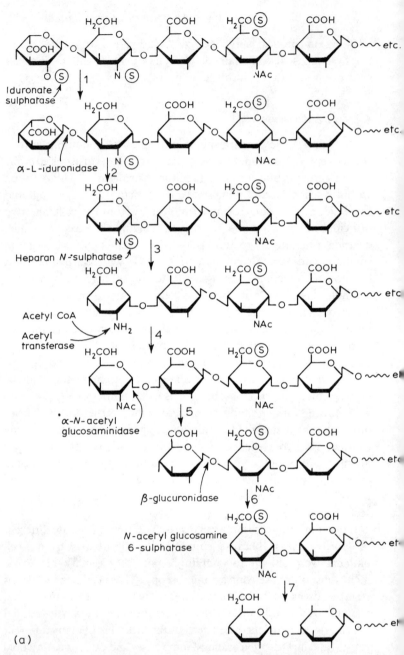

Fig. 4.1 (a) The basic structure of the mucopolysaccharide heparan sulphate consisting of chains of uronic acid glucosamine residues. The former may be glucuronic acid or iduronic acid which is either sulphated or unsulphated. The amino group of the latter may be sulphated or acetylated with an additional sulphation on the hydroxyl group in the 6 position. A

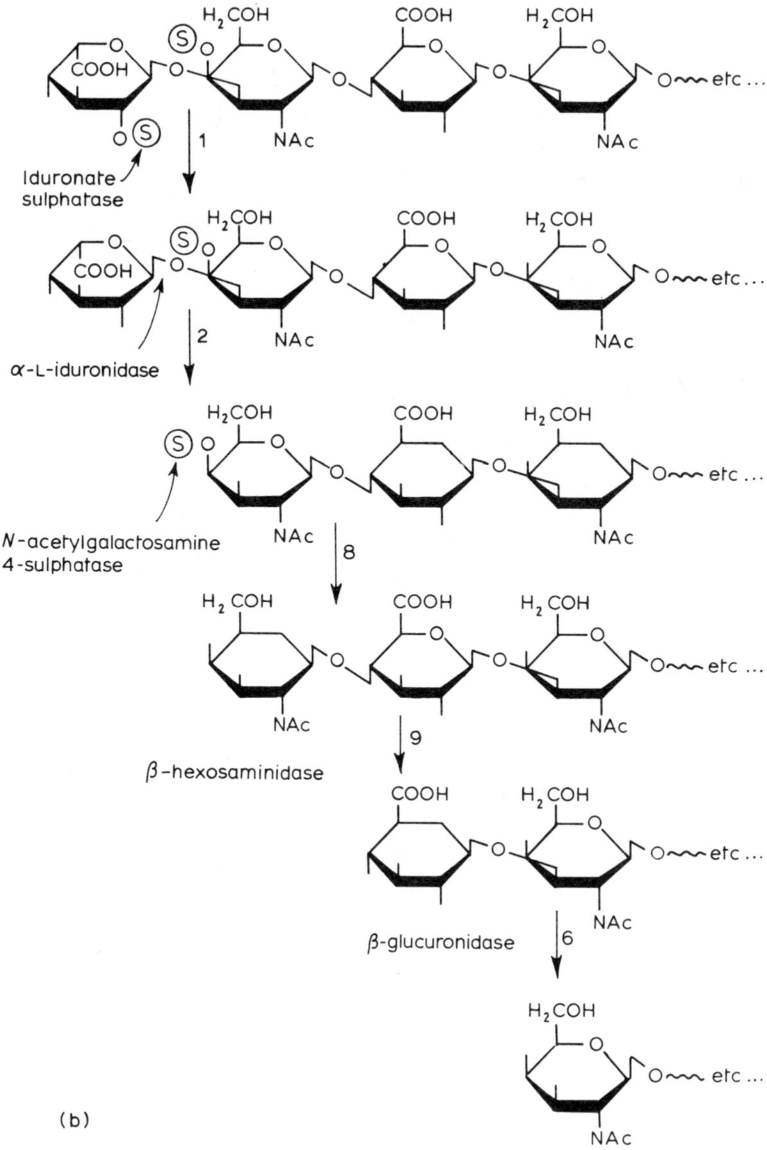

Iduronate
sulphatase

α-L-iduronidase

N-acetylgalactosamine
4-sulphatase

β-hexosaminidase

β-glucuronidase

(b)

series of enzymes degrade the molecule and inherited defects of all of these are known, causing accumulation of the mucopolysaccharide residues in tissues and excretion in the urine. The deficiency of Hurler syndrome (see Section 4.2.2) is enzyme 2, α-L-iduronidase. (b) The structure of dermatan sulphate which consists of chains of uronic acid and sulphated N-acetylgalactosamine residues. The uronic acid may be glucuronic acid or sulphated or unsulphated L-iduronic acid. Deficiency diseases are known for all the steps in the degradative pathway, enzyme 2 being the defect in Hurler syndrome.

(c) The degradative pathway of keratan sulphate. This mucopolysaccharide contains sulphated or unsulphated galactose residues alternating with *N*-acetylglucosamine. Defects in this pathway exist, but since it does not involve the enzyme α-L-iduronidase, keratan sulphate is not accumulated in Hurler syndrome.

plasma levels of the corresponding enzymes. In addition, the culture medium in which hydrolase deficient fibroblasts were grown contained high concentrations of the enzymes. These findings suggested that the affected hydrolases were being lost from the cell, rather than localized within the lysosomes.

Further experiments on the mechanism of the distribution defect in I-cell disease implied that the abnormality occurred in the enzymes themselves rather than within the lysosomes, because it was observed that hexosaminidase B and cathepsin from normal people were taken up at the usual rate by the lysosomes of I-cell patients, whereas the same enzymes derived from patients were not accumulated by normal lysosomes. The defect in the I-cell enzymes was traced to the mannose phosphate residues within them which normally function as identity markers, directing the enzyme to be taken up by the lysosomes. In the abnormal hexosaminidase and cathepsin, the identity markers tended to be in the dephosphorylated form.

The post-translational modification of the primary peptides of the hydrolases, to add the identity markers, occurs in the endoplasmic reticulum in two steps: firstly the mannose molecules are added; secondly, the mannose is phosphorylated. Presumably the second reaction is at fault in I-cell disease.

The phosphorylation of mannose involves the formation of a diester intermediate in which mannose is linked through a phosphate to N-acetylglucosamine (Fig. 4.2). N-acetylglucosamine is then split from the diester leaving a mannose-6-phosphate residue on the protein, but the activity of this specific N-acetylglucosaminidase is normal in I-cell fibroblasts. There is evidence, however, that the formation of the diester is defective in the patients. It is probable that

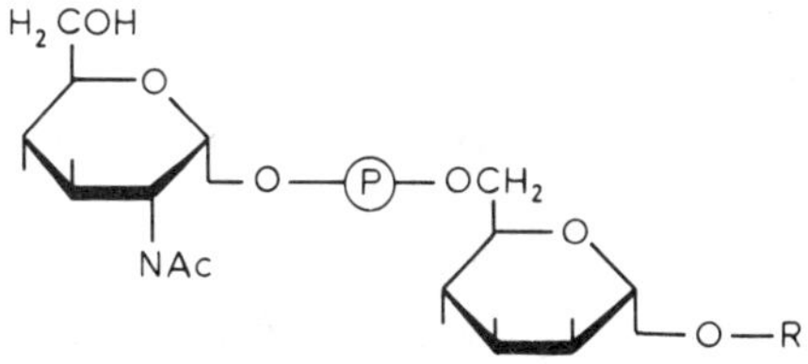

Fig. 4.2 Structure of the phosphodiester N-acetylglucosamine-l-phosphate-6-mannose, intermediate in the synthesis of the mannose phosphate recognition marker. R represents the oligosaccharide on the newly synthesized acid hydrolases with six to eight mannose residues.

the synthesis of the diester on the mannosylated enzyme requires UDPN-acetylglucosamine as cofactor and that it is the enzyme which catalyses this reaction which is abnormal in I-cell patients.

4.3   Pathogenic mechanisms related to derangement of cellular metabolism

4.3.1   Deficient end product

An important consequence of an inherited enzyme defect may be failure to produce the end-product of the metabolic pathway (see Fig. 1.2(d)). However, it should be appreciated that a deficiency of the end-product does not necessarily occur: partial activity of the enzyme, together with a higher substrate concentration caused by accumulation of precursors, often results in normal, or near normal, synthesis of the end-product. This situation has been referred to as a 'leaky' mutation. Another possibility is that there is an alternative source of the product. For example, in phenylketonuria (Section 3.3), tyrosine cannot be made from phenylalanine and it becomes an essential amino acid. However, tyrosine deficiency is not usually a problem in phenylketonuria because the amino acid is a constituent of all dietary proteins.

Reference has already been made in Section 1.1 to albinism, in which the end-product of the melanin synthetic pathways, in the melanocyte, is not produced. This leads to a lack of pigmentation and, thus, to light sensitivity of the skin and eyes, which is an unpleasant feature of the condition. There are, in fact, two melanins responsible for skin pigmentation. One, eumelanin is brown/black in colour, the other, pheomelanin, is a red/yellow pigment. The pathways for synthesis of both melanins are shown in Fig. 4.3. The usual cause of albinism is a partial, or complete, deficiency of tyrosinase, which catalyses two steps which are common to the metabolic pathways of both pigments.

A second example of a disorder in which the lack of formation of an end-product is important is the glycogen storage disease due to liver glucose-6-phosphatase deficiency. Alternative names for the condition are glycogen storage disease type 1 and Von Gierke's disease. Figure 4.4 illustrates the unique role of glucose-6-phosphatase in releasing glucose from the liver for transport to other organs, via

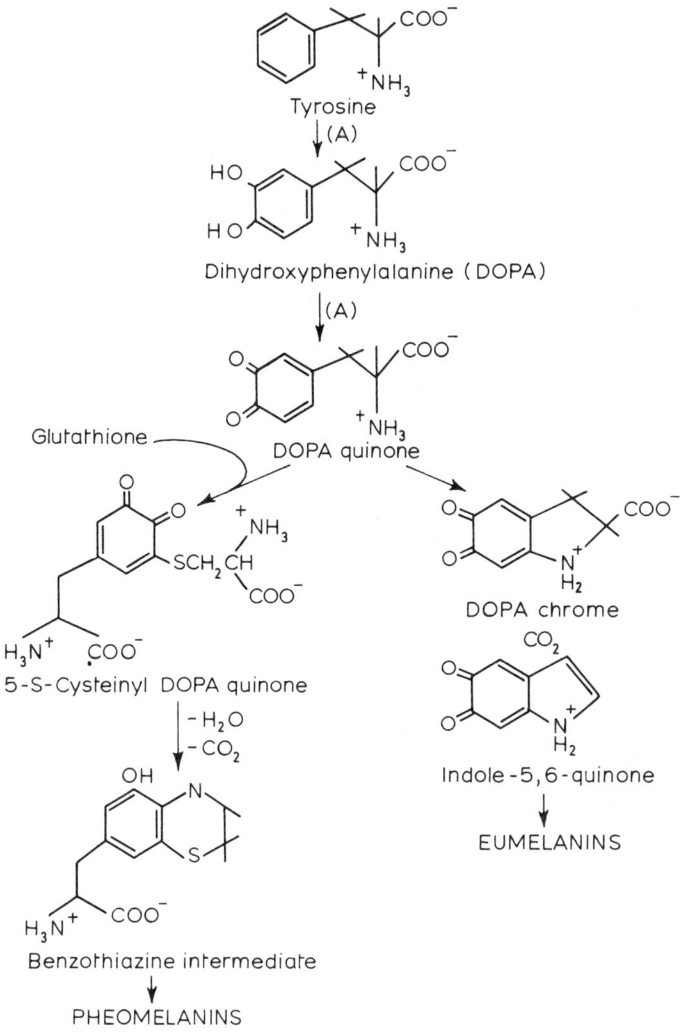

Fig. 4.3 Pathways for synthesis of eumelanins and pheomelanins. Enzyme A, tyrosinase, is common to both pathways and is deficient in albinism.

the blood circulation. The enzyme catalyses the last stage, which is common to two major metabolic pathways for generating glucose; namely from glycogen, through glucose-1-phosphate, and from gluconeogenesis. As the liver is the only organ which is able to release glucose into the blood stream in the fasting state, the patient with glucose-6-phosphatase deficiency is liable to very profound

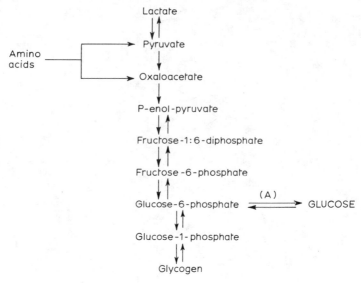

Fig. 4.4   Metabolic pathways related to the glucose-6-phosphatase defect. Enzyme A is glucose-6-phosphatase.

hypoglycaemia, if not fed regularly. Apart from this inability to make the glucose end-product, the precursor glycogen accumulates, which is the reason for the name glycogen storage disease.

Other diseases in which the clinical features can be directly related to the absence of an end-product are those in which the affected enzyme is in the synthetic pathway of a hormone, or of the active form of a vitamin cofactor. The clinical picture in these circumstances is that associated with the specific hormone deficiency, more commonly caused by a gross glandular abnormality, or a vitamin deficiency, seen usually as a result of nutritional inadequacy. Examples of this phenomenon are, firstly, the diseases affecting the production of thyroxine by the thyroid gland. The synthesis of thyroxine and its abnormalities are shown in Fig. 4.5. These subtle causes of hypothyroidism are clinically indistinguishable from those which occur more commonly in newborn infants, either from a congenital absence, or the possession of a non-viable, thyroid gland. Secondly, the failure to produce the active cofactor forms of vitamin B_{12} may produce metabolic abnormalities similar to those found in vitamin deficient states. Methylmalonic aciduria, due to defective synthesis of adenosyl cobalamin, has already been discussed (Section 3.3.2).

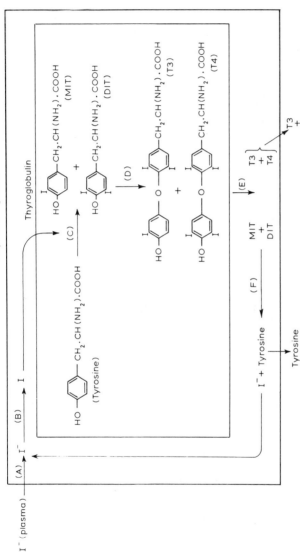

Fig. 4.5 Synthesis of thyroxin within the thyroid gland. The stages of the synthesis, at which inherited defects are known, are as follows: (A), uptake of inorganic iodide into the gland; (B), conversion of iodide ion to elemental iodine by peroxidase; (C), iodination of tyrosine to the iodotyrosines, within the thyroglobulin molecule; (D), the coupling of the iodotyrosines to tri-iodothyronine (T3) and thyroxin (T4); (E), The release of T3 and T4 and the uncoupled iodotyrosines from thyroglobulin; (F), the deiodination of released iodotyrosines causing unnecessary iodine loss and deficiency.

4.3.2 *Precursor accumulation*

The accumulation of metabolites prior to a metabolic block (see Fig. 1.2(c)) is regarded as the likely cause of the pathological changes associated with many disorders. The rationale of most tentative treatments of the inherited diseases is to prevent this accumulation from occurring and this approach has had frequent success. Occasionally a clinical sign can be explained directly by the raised metabolite level; for example, the acidosis of methylmalonic acidaemia is due to the excess of methylmalonic and propionic acids (Section 2.2.2). In other cases it is reasonably assumed that there is a link between an increased percursor concentration and the pathology of a condition. The accumulation of macromolecules in the storage diseases is presumed to be the direct cause of the generalized cellular damage which occurs in some affected organs. In other diseases in which metabolite accumulation is thought to be part of the pathology the mechanisms are merely speculative and the subject of experimental observation. Two typical examples of this situation will be considered.

In phenylketonuria (Section 3.3), the most important symptom is severe mental retardation. However, the risk of this most distressing feature is virtually abolished by a dietary restriction of phenylalanine, to reduce the body pool of the amino acid to near normal levels. The way in which phenylalanine excess causes brain damage has stimulated much experimental work. The main hypothesis behind most of this work is that phenylalanine interferes with normal myelin synthesis. This originated from the findings of widespread deficiency of myelin in the brains of phenylketonuric patients, at postmortem.

Myelin forms a protective sheath around nerve fibres and it is essential for the correct functioning of the axons. It makes up a large proportion of brain mass, particularly the white matter, and it consists of a basic protein, together with phospholipid and cholesterol. It is critical for normal brain growth that the rate of myelin synthesis is appropriate for the particular phase of development and that it is assembled correctly round the nerve fibres. It is probable that the myelin deficiency of phenylketonuria is due to interference with normal synthesis, rather than later demyelination, because the rate at which brain damage occurs at any given age is directly related to the normal rate of myelination at that time. Thus the greatest loss of intellectual capacity occurs in the early months of life, when brain development is greatest.

The two principal explanations for the interference with myelin formation in phenylketonuria suppose that it is the synthesis of the basic protein which is affected. The first postulates that high circulating levels of phenylalanine inhibit the transport of other amino acids into the brain. There is reasonable evidence from observations in phenylketonuric patients, and in experimental animals, that excess phenylalanine does affect the normal transport and distribution of other amino acids. Thus, the amino acids are in a state of imbalance in the brain and this will lead to abnormal protein synthesis. Alternatively it is possible that a specific deficiency of tryptophan inhibits protein synthesis, because the inadequacy of this amino acid in experimental systems causes a disaggregation of polysomes. The second mechanism suggests a direct effect of a high phenylalanine on protein synthesis. It has been shown experimentally that this could occur at two stages:

(1) The charging of transfer RNA with the correct amino acids.
(2) Inhibition of translation initiation. It has been possible to demonstrate inhibition of neural protein synthesis by phenylalanine, probably due to a reduction in the availability of the translation initiator, met-tRNA.

The other example of the experimental approach to pathogenesis is the disorders of galactose metabolism. Galactose epimerase deficiency has already been referred to in Section 3.4.3. The most important disorder of galactose metabolism, however, is due to a deficiency of galactose-1-phosphate uridyl transferase (transferase – enzyme B in Fig. 3.9) and, finally, galactokinase deficiency (enzyme C in Fig. 3.9) has been described. The first two of these disorders are much more severe in their clinical presentation than galactokinase deficiency, which is almost benign. In particular, the serious diseases are associated with damage to the liver.

It has always been considered that the metabolite which causes the severe pathology in the galactose disorders is galactose-1-phosphate. This conclusion is consistent with the fact that galactose-1-phosphate accumulates in transferase and epimerase deficiencies, but not in galactokinase deficiency. It should be noted that UDPGal is also increased in epimerase deficiency and it is unique in this respect (Fig. 4.6). It appears that UDPGal is the first compound to

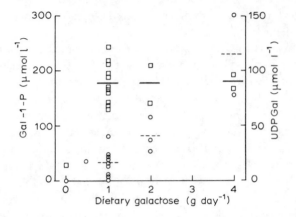

Fig. 4.6 Accumulation of metabolites in a child with uridine diphosphate galactose-4-epimerase defect on varying galactose intakes. ∘, level of Gal-1-P in packed red cells; ----, mean level of Gal-1-P for samples taken at the same galactose intake; □, level of UDPGal in packed red cells; —, mean level of UDPGal for samples taken at the same galactose intake.

accumulate in epimerase deficiency when only small amounts of galactose are being metabolized, presumably because galactose-1-phosphate can be removed by transferase reaction, using UDPGlc which has been newly synthesized by the pyrophosphorylase reaction:

$$UTP + Glc\text{-}1\text{-}P \longrightarrow UDPGlc + PP$$

However, as more galactose is metabolized the availability of UDPGlc becomes limiting, in the absence of epimerase to regenerate it from UDPGal, and galactose-1-phosphate will now accumulate.

The toxic effects of galactose-1-phosphate have usually been explained by its inhibition of various other enzymes, phosphoglucomutase, for example, However, although inhibition of phosphoglucomutase occurs in isolated enzyme systems, it cannot be demonstrated *in vivo* with experimental animal studies, nor with galactosaemic cells in tissue culture. This has led to an alternative hypothesis, to explain liver damage in particular, in which the depletion of UTP is the critical factor.

There is good experimental evidence that depletion of the high energy uridyl compound in hepatic cells inhibits their growth and, eventually, causes cell death. The cell damage in galactosaemia remains related to the accumulation of galactose-1-phosphate, insofar as it traps high energy phosphate, without the normal conversion of galactose to glucose. This restricts the availability of ATP for UTP synthesis. Moreover, the accumulation of UDPGal, which occurs in the early stages of galactose metabolism in epimerase deficiency, is extremely energy dependent, requiring 3 mol of ATP to metabolize 1 mol of galactose to UDPGal, as shown below:

$$
\begin{array}{ll}
\text{Gal} + \text{ATP} & \longrightarrow \text{Gal-1-P} + \text{ADP} \\
\text{UMP} + 2\text{ATP} & \longrightarrow \text{UTP} + 2\text{ADP} \\
\text{UTP} + \text{Glc-1-P} & \longrightarrow \text{UDPGlc} + \text{PP} \\
\text{Gal-1-P} + \text{UDPGlc} & \longrightarrow \text{UDPGal} + \text{Glc-1-P} \\
\hline
\text{Gal} + \text{UMP} + 3\text{ATP} & \longrightarrow \text{UDPGal} + 3\text{ADP} + \text{PP}
\end{array}
$$

This may explain the fact that the liver of an epimerase deficiency patient appeared to be extremely sensitive to small amounts of dietary galactose, reacting much more rapidly than transferase deficient patients in the same situation.

4.3.3   Abnormal metabolites

Figure 1.2(d) illustrates how some of the accumulated substances preceding the enzyme block in a metabolic pathway may be diverted into the synthesis of one, or more, abnormal metabolites. Usually it is not strictly correct to call them abnormal metabolites; but a pathway of very minor significance, in normal circumstances, takes a greater importance. A few examples will illustrate how the production of large amounts of a normally minor metabolite may have pathological results.

Primary oxaluria is an autosomal recessive disease which is associated with renal stones. Stone formation may occur at a very early age. The stones are composed of calcium oxalate and the cause of their formation is an increased urinary excretion of oxalate, about three to ten times the highest level found in a normal person. It has been established that plasma oxalate is also raised, although very varied results have been obtained because of the poor analytical methods available.

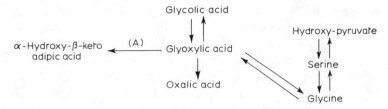

Fig. 4.7 Pathways of oxalate production. Enzyme A, α-ketoglutarate: glyoxylate carboligase, is deficient in hyperoxaluria type I.

Normally about 500μmol of oxalate are excreted per day. This is derived from several sources including the diet, the metabolism of ascorbic acid and synthesis from glycine and glycolic acid via a pathway shown in Fig. 4.7. It is probable that the last of these sources is of minor importance in normal circumstances. However, in the most common type of primary oxaluria, an enzyme block at point A (α-ketoglutarate: glyoxylate carboligase) diverts the pathway into producing vastly increased amounts of oxalate. The body pool of glycolic acid and glyoxylic acid are increased also.

A further example of the pathological role of an abnormal metabolite is afforded by the galactose disorders (see Fig. 3.9). Both transferase and galactokinase deficiency are known to cause very early cataracts. Since galactose is the only common precursor, and accumulates in both these disorders it would appear that the cataract formation is related to this. However, it is now established that the actual cause of the cataracts is a metabolite, galactitol, which is formed from galactose by the enzyme aldose reductase.

When the galactose concentration is increased, galactitol synthesis can occur within the eye lens and, once formed, the metabolite diffuses from the eye extremely slowly. As it accumulates, it causes an osmotic swelling of the lens and a disruption of lens fibres. Although many other changes are found during cataract formation, there is no doubt that the accumulation of glactitol is the primary defect. If the synthesis of galactitol is inhibited, or the osmotic swelling is prevented, the formation of cataracts will not proceed.

There has been much work, experimental and largely hypothetical, on the contribution of abnormal phenylalanine metabolites to the clinical defect of phenylketonuria. As one example of this work, phenylpyruvic acid, phenyllactic acid and phenylacetic acid (Fig. 3.5.) have been shown to be potent inhibitors of the enzymes which decarboxylate dihydroxy-phenylalanine, 5-hydroxytryptophane

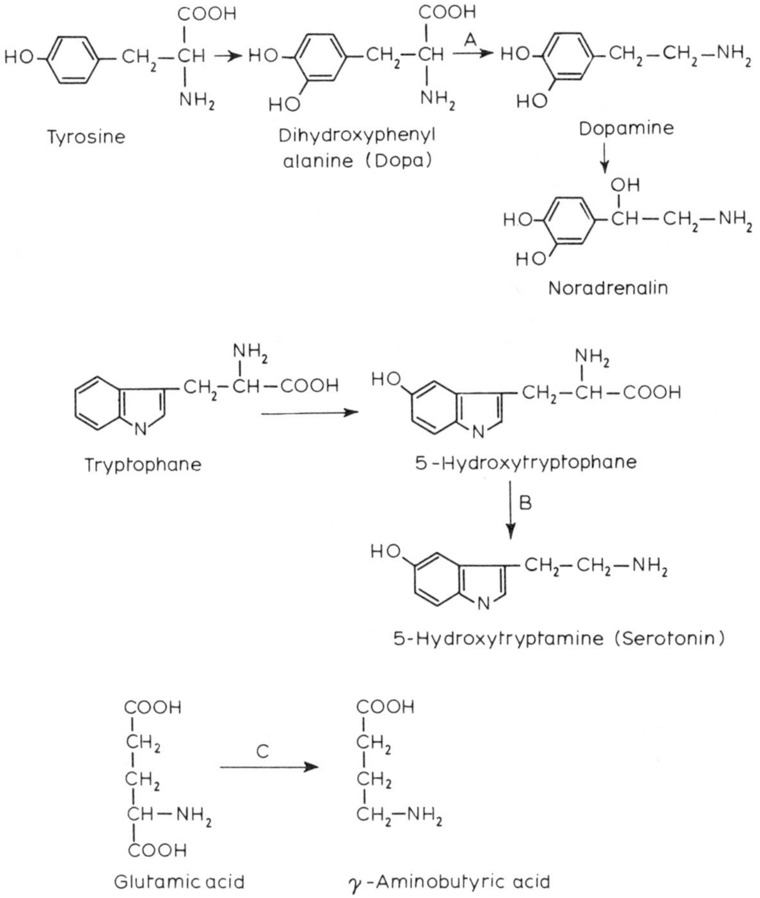

Fig. 4.8 Pathways for the synthesis of catecholamines (noradrenalin), serotonin and γ-aminobutyric acid. A, B and C are the decarboxylase steps.

and glutamate, leading to the synthesis of catecholamines, 5-hydroxytryptamine (serotonin) and γ-aminobutyric acid, respectively (Fig. 4.8). Catecholamines and serotonin function in the central nervous system and in peripheral nerves as neurotransmitters, whereas γ-aminobutyric acid is a neuro-inhibitor. A failure to synthesize the correct amounts of these substances would lead to far reaching neurological sequelae.

There is some indication that the inhibition of decarboxylases demonstrated *in vitro*, does occur in phenylketonuria. In untreated patients, plasma adrenalin and platelet serotonin levels are depressed. Although there is no certainty that the substances are deficient in nervous tissue, decarboxylase inhibitors can be shown to depress the concentration of the amines in the brains of animals.

Since the inhibition of the decarboxylases would appear to be completely reversible on treating the phenylketonuric patient with a low phenylalanine diet, it is not clear that the 'mono-amine' hypothesis can offer an explanation for the permanent brain damage which occurs if treatment is not begun soon after birth. The demyelination hypothesis seems to offer a much better explanation of this aspect of the disease. This does not imply that the mono-amine hypothesis is unimportant. It is well documented that the behaviour of phenylketonuric patients deteriorates when phenylalanine levels are uncontrolled and the mood changes have been correlated with depression of platelet serotonin levels. It is possible that a depression of brain amines affects behaviour; this may lead to learning difficulties which could have a permanent effect on intellectual development.

4.3.4 *Metabolic abnormalities complicated by feedback control in the pathway*

Figure 4.9 shows how the consequences of an enzyme defect may be exaggerated by an effect on a controlling step in a metabolic pathway. The rate of formation of end-product (D) may be sensitively controlled if there is feedback inhibition on an earlier, rate limiting, step in its synthetic pathway (at enzyme[a]). This negative feedback

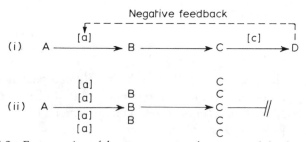

Fig. 4.9 Exaggeration of the consequences of an enzyme defect by an effect on a controlling step of a metabolic pathway: in (i) the metabolic pathway is controlled by the end-product D exerting negative feedback on the activity of the rate limiting enzyme [a]; When the end-product is no longer formed (ii) due to a defect in enzyme [c], negative feedback control is no longer applied, [a] increases in concentration and/or activity, and B and C accumulate in very large amounts.

may be achieved by end-product inhibition of the controlling enzyme, or repression of synthesis of this enzyme. If there is a defect in the pathway, leading to lack of formation of D, the control of the pathway would be lost and precursors would tend to accumulate in particularly large quantities.

The pathogenesis of a group of disorders known as the porphyrias, which are defects in the synthetic pathway of haem (Fig. 4.10) is believed to involve, in part, a failure of negative feedback control. Acute intermittent porphyria (AIP) is one specific porphyria, in which the deficient enzyme is porphobilinogen deaminase (alternatively known as uroporphyrinogen synthase). AIP is inherited as a dominant characteristics, although only about one third of the heterozygotes, who can be shown to have about 50% activity of the

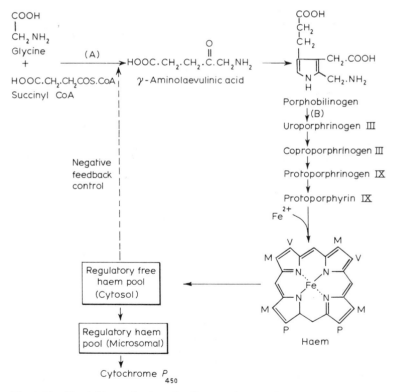

Fig. 4.10 Haem biosynthesis and utilization for cytochrome P_{450} synthesis. Enzyme A is γ-aminolaevulinic acid synthetase. Enzyme B is porphobilinogen deaminase which is affected in acute intermittent porphyria.

deaminase in red cells, liver and cultured skin fibroblasts, appear to suffer any clinical abnormality.

Individuals with AIP who are clinically affected, have severe attacks of abdominal pain, neurological and mental disturbances and muscle weakness. These acute episodes are precipitated by drugs, particularly barbiturates and oestrogens, and by other factors, including a low calorie diet. The attacks are accompanied by a vast excretion of porphyrin precursors, γ-aminolaevulinic acid (ALA) and porphobilinogen (PBG), whereas these compounds are normal, or only marginally abnormal, in a quiescent phase. The common determinant of the clinical symptoms appears to be an acute disturbance of the autonomic nervous system and an hypothesis attributes this to ALA and PBG acting as inhibitors of neurotransmission. However, this is not absolutely proven.

A disruption of normal haem synthesis control is implicated in the over production of ALA and PBG and in the acute attacks of AIP. It is well established that the ALA synthetase is the rate limiting enzyme in the pathway and negative feedback control is believed to be exerted on this enzyme by a regulatory free haem pool in the mitochondrion, most probably by repression of enzyme synthesis.

In normal circumstances the amount of the porphyrin precursors produced can be metabolized completely by individuals who have only 50% activity of PBG deaminase, and no accumulation occurs. The synthesis of haem is also normal. It is suggested that this equilibrium is disturbed by drugs requiring cytochrome P_{450} for their metabolism, and which induce the synthesis of the apoprotein of the cytochrome. The apoprotein then chelates haem from the free haem pool; this derepresses the synthesis of ALA synthetase, which allows a large flux of ALA and PBG to be formed. The deficient PBG deaminase cannot metabolize the increased amount of porphyrin precursors. They will then accumulate, and are excreted in large quantities.

4.4 Disorders of membrane function

Many inherited disorders may be explained by defects in membrane function and are caused by a change in the structure of a specific protein which is an essential component of the particular membrane mechanism that is abnormal. Inherited abnormalities in membrane function may be divided into three types.

4.4.1 Mechanisms for the transfer of small molecules

Small molecules may have an active transport process for transferring them across a membrane. These transport mechanisms have a degree of specificity which is believed to be determined by the protein constituent of the membrane; although, as will be seen later, the specificity is sometimes much broader than that usually associated with enzyme reactions. A mutation in the structure of a transport protein may render the system completely inactive, or may change its specificity.

Many examples of transport disorders involving the renal tubular membrane have been recognized, affecting the movement of various inorganic ions, monosaccharides and amino acids. The result of this sort of defect is that the particular low molecular weight substance, or substances, will not be reabsorbed from the glomerular filtrate and there will be excessive urinary loss. This may cause profound metabolic and clinical disorder. Amino acid transport mechanisms have been investigated in some depth and will be considered here.

There appears to be a close similarity between the transport mechanisms for the readsorption of amino acids in the renal tubule and for their absorption by the intestine. In many cases inherited disorders affect both processes simultaneously. The bulk of amino acid transport within the intestine is achieved by transport systems with a very broad specificity, called 'group transport systems'. These have a low K_m and a very high capacity for the movement of amino acids. Many amino acids may use the same system and must have similar physicochemical properties. Five transport systems have been described with the following broad specificity:

(1) The dicarboxylic amino acids: aspartic acid, glutamic acid.
(2) The basic amino acids and cystine: ornithine, lysine, arginine and cystine.
(3) The imino acids and glycine: proline, hydroxyproline and glycine.
(4) The neutral amino acids: glycine, alanine, serine, threonine, leucine, iso-leucine, valine, phenylalanine, tyrosine, tryptophan, histidine.
(5) β-amino acids: β-alanine.

The group transport systems are not the only means of transporting amino acids. Mechanisms have been demonstrated which are specific for one amino acid, although in general they have a relatively low capacity. In addition, it is possible to transport dipeptides across the intestinal wall. The alternative methods for the transport of amino acids explains why a defect in one system does not produce a profound depletion of the affected amino acids. Figure 4.11 shows diagrammatically various transport systems in the proximal tubule for the imino acids, glycine and other neutral amino acids.

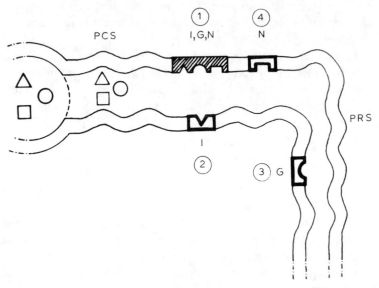

Fig. 4.11 Amino acid transport sites on the proximal nephron. PCS, proximal convoluted segment; PRS, pars recta segment; (1), a shared high capacity, low affinity site for imino acids (I), glycine (G) and the neutral amino acids (N); (2), a specific low capacity, high affinity carrier site for the imino acids; (3), a specific low capacity, high affinity site for glycine; (4), a site for neutral amino acid transport. Imino-glycinuria probably involves a mutation at site (1) and Hartnup disease at site (4).

Inherited abnormalities occur most frequently in the group transport systems. Since these presumably represent a structural defect in the protein component of the transport mechanism, it is easy to understand that the disorders may be very heterogeneous. In some cases the transport system may become completely inactive, in others it may be partially active. On the other hand the broad specificity may be changed and certain amino acids may become preferentially transported.

There are three, well-established disorders of group transport.

(*a*) *Cystinuria*

Cystinuria was one of Garrod's original inborn errors of metabolism (Section 1.1), but some 50 years later it was discovered that not only cystine, but also ornithine, lysine and arginine, were excreted in excessive amounts by the patient. Moreover, none of the amino acids appeared to accumulate within the body. These findings were not consistent with Garrod's initial interpretation of cystinuria as a metabolic defect. Subsequent work showed that the disease could be explained by an abnormality in the group transport system for the basic amino acids and cystine in the renal tubule, causing increased loss of all four amino acids in the urine. However, it also became apparent that the same amino acids were absorbed poorly from the intestine, also indicating an inherited abnormality in the intestinal transport system.

The defect in cystinuria is clearly heterogeneous and at least three structural forms of the transport protein are indicated. The three allelic forms of the gene may be differentiated by a combination of two factors. First is the degree to which the amino aciduria occurs in heterozygotes in the same family. Secondly, by studying the defect in small intestinal biopsy samples taken from the homozygous patient.

(*b*) *Hartnup disease*

Hartnup disease is another, clearly distinguished, clinical condition, due to a defect in the neutral amino acid transport system. There is a marked amino aciduria which may involve all the substances handled by the neutral group transport mechanism, and intestinal absorption of these amino acids is also affected. One clinical feature of patients with Hartnup disease is short stature. This is attributed to a relative deficiency of neutral amino acids, particularly those which are essential. The deficiency of essential amino acid may have been more critical were it not for the intestinal absorption of dipeptides, mentioned earlier.

The more serious symptoms of Hartnup disease, however, are an intermittent, pellagra type, rash, cerebellar ataxia and a variety of psychiatric features. These are caused by a deficiency of nicotinamide, which is usually synthesized from tryptophane, one of the amino acids that is poorly absorbed in the disorder. Once the problem is diagnosed, the symptoms may be alleviated very simply by the administration of oral nicotinamide.

(c) *Imino-glycinuria*

As the name suggests; imino-glycinuria is a defect in the transport system for imino acids and glycine. Proline, hydroxyproline and glycine are present in the urine in larger amounts than normal. The condition does not seem to cause any harmful effects.

4.4.2 *The transfer of macromolecules*

Large molecules cross the cell membrane by a very different process to that of small molecules. It is known as endocytosis. First, macro-molecules bind to a cell surface receptor protein which, as usual, confers a specificity to the process. Once the molecule is bound it is trapped by the membrane invaginating into the cell. Ultimately, this portion of membrane breaks away to form a separate endocytic vesicle which contains the macromolecule. The macromolecule is transported in the cell by the vesicle and may eventually be degraded within it.

One form of inherited hyperlipidaemia is caused as a direct consequence of a defect in a membrane receptor. This is the receptor for low density lipoprotein (LDL). Because of the membrane defect normal cellular degradation of apo-LDL does not occur and, there-fore, it accumulates in plasma with its bound lipid moiety, mostly cholesterol. Thus patients with this particular inherited disease have high plasma cholesterol levels. This results in lipid deposition in arterial walls and serious arterial disease.

4.4.3 *Hormone receptors*

Many peptide hormones exert their effects on cell metabolism without actually entering the cell. They act by binding to specific membrane receptors on the cell surface. Their effect is then transmitted across the membrane through a stimulation of adenylate cyclase activity, which causes the formation of cyclic AMP in the cell and this produces the desired regulation of cell metabolism. The mechanism of adenylate cyclase activation has been studied in detail and is more complex than originally thought. A schematic repre-sentation of the process involving parathyroid hormone (PTH) is shown in Fig. 4.12.

PTH binds to a receptor at the cell surface to form a freely

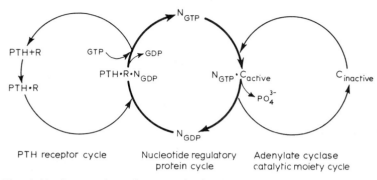

Fig. 4.12 Proposed mechanism of adenylate cyclase activation. PTH, parathyroid hormone; R, receptor; N, nucleotide regulatory protein; C, catalytic moiety; GTP, guanine triphosphate; GDP, guanine diphosphate. See Section 4.4.3 for further explanation of the diagram.

reversible complex. This induces a conformational change in the receptor which causes it to bind with a guanine nucleotide containing regulatory protein (N–protein). The binding of PTH–receptor complex to the N–protein results in a loss of GDP from the protein, and a consequential binding of GTP to the nucleotide site on the regulatory protein. At this point hormone receptor complex splits off from the N-protein which is now primed with GTP. The N–protein–GTP complex interacts with the 'catalytic moiety', forming active adenylate cyclase and the synthesis of cyclic AMP from ATP. During this action phosphate is lost and the components revert to inactive catalytic moiety and GDP bound to regulatory N–protein.

Patients with the disease known as pseudohypoparathyroidism have all the clinical signs of parathyroid hormone deficiency, including hypocalcaemia and hyperphosphataemia, but have increased circulating levels of the hormone. It is postulated that they have an end organ defect affecting the action of PTH on kidney, and possibly bone. Studies of patients with this inherited defect suggest that the precise location of the defect within the scheme described for PTH action may vary. However, a proportion of patients have been found in which there is a deficiency of regulatory N–protein and this is presumed to be the primary protein change in these cases.

5

Diagnosis of inherited metabolic diseases

5.1 Introduction

One of the main objectives of the medical investigation of a patient must be to make a diagnosis. In the case of the inherited metabolic diseases there is a distinct advantage that a very specific diagnosis may be made with great certainty. The practical importance of making a firm diagnosis is as follows:

(1) It should give clear indications of the correct course of management of the patient. For example, there may be an established treatment for the disease or, if the circumstances justify it, a prenatal diagnosis early in a pregnancy may allow the selective abortion of an affected fetus.

(2) It may enable the clinician to give an accurate prognosis. However, the clinical heterogeneity of many diseases has already been stressed and, therefore, the prediction of future developments may sometimes be difficult.

(3) It allows clear counselling of parents regarding the risks of a recurrence of a disease in future pregnancies.

In this chapter the broad principles of diagnosis will be discussed first, followed by a consideration of the application of these principles to three diagnostic procedures; namely, the most common situation in which tests are initiated by the suspicions of a clinician, biochemical diagnostic screening of a whole newborn population and prenatal diagnosis of pregnancies known to be at risk of producing an affected child.

5.2 General principles of biochemical diagnosis

Inherited metabolic diseases may now be diagnosed at three levels of expression; at the gene level, at the level of the primary phenotypic change, i.e. the enzyme, and at the level of the metabolic changes.

5.2.1 The gene

It has been possible for several years to detect variations, or polymorphisms, within a particular DNA sequence of interest. This technology has been applied to the diagnosis of many abnormalities of haemoglobin synthesis. Essentially, it may be used to determine the genotype of any new member of a family known to be at risk for a particular disorder providing there has been a detailed study of the index case and close relations. It is very suitable for prenatal diagnosis. Applications of the technique to metabolic diseases are only just appearing.

The 'diagnostic' polymorphisms may occur in a number of places in the DNA sequence. Ideally it would be sited in the coding sequence of the gene which is affected in the disease. In this situation one is examining the actual nucleotide change which is causing abnormal protein synthesis. However, this situation is not often achieved. Many polymorphisms occur throughout the long DNA sequences which are not necessary for coding a protein. These may be of little significance, but this is immaterial with regard to present considerations. It is only necessary to be able to recognize one specific polymorphism in the DNA sequence which is invariably associated with the abnormal gene during meiosis. It is also required that the normal gene is never linked to this particular polymorphism.

The detection of polymorphisms in DNA structure is achieved principally by the use of enzymes which split the molecule at points with specific nucleotide sequences, thus fragmenting the DNA chain. These enzymes, many hundred of which are known, are called restriction endonucleases. The fragments of double-stranded DNA produced may have 'staggered' or 'blunt' ends depending on the sequence recognized. For example, the endonuclease known as EcoR1 will split guanine from adenine when they occur in the sequence GAATTC, where G, A, T and C are guanine adenine, thymine and cytosine respectively.

This enzyme will produce a staggered split as follows:

```
G  |        AATTC
   |____
        |
  CTTAA |  G
```

On the other hand, the enzyme Sma 1 cleaves G and C in the sequence CCC GGG. It produces a blunt ended split:

```
CCC  |  GGG

GGG  |  CCC
```

The object is to find a restriction endonuclease which splits the DNA sequence at the point where the critical polymorphism occurs. In this situation, when DNA containing the polymorphism is incubated with the restriction endonuclease it will produce different length fragments to those obtained with the DNA associated with the normal gene. The technique by which the polymorphisms are detected has led to them being called restriction fragment length polymorphisms (RFLPs).

The different sized nucleotide fragments may be separated by gel electrophoresis and it is important to be able to easily recognize the change in the critical fragment which indicates the polymorphism. To do this the fragments are usually transferred or 'blotted' onto a nitrocellulose sheet and then a radioactive labelled DNA probe is used which hybridizes on the nitrocellulose sheet with the fragments one is interested in. Thus it is possible to detect the 'normal' fragment and, also, the 'abnormal' fragment which will have an altered electrophoretic mobility. In most situations the polymorphism will be near to the gene and the DNA probe used will be the gene, or part of the gene, which is being investigated. Figure 5.1 shows how the process will work when both the normal fragment and abnormal fragment signalling the RFLP contain the gene sequence.

The advantages of DNA techniques are that it should be possible to make a diagnosis on any nucleated cell, even though the gene concerned may not be expressed in that cell. The disadvantage is that one restriction endonuclease, indicating one particular RFLP, will only be applicable in a proportion of families with a disease. Recent work on phenylketonuria has shown that three restriction enzymes will enable the detection of the abnormal gene in 75% of families with the disease. Work on phenylketonuria is particularly important since the enzyme which is affected in the disorder is only present in

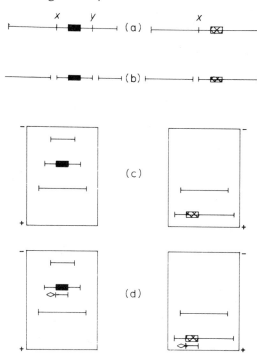

Fig. 5.1 Detection of DNA polymorphisms associated with a normal gene ■ and its mutant form ⊠. The normal gene is associated with two restriction sites at x and y, whereas y is absent from the DNA sequence containing the mutant gene (a). On treatment with the appropriate restriction endonuclease completely different DNA fragments are formed (b), which separate and give different patterns on electrophoresis (c). The gene probe ⊶ hybridizes with fragments of different size and electrophoretic mobility in subjects possessing the normal, or mutant, gene (d).

the liver, making diagnosis by enzyme assay very difficult.

5.2.2 The enzyme

Estimating the level of the affected enzyme may provide an excellent means of making a diagnosis, providing biological material is readily available in which the particular enzyme is normally present and in which the deficiency is also expressed. An accurate and precise method of enzyme assay must be available. Figure 5.2 gives the results of red cell transferase assays in the diagnosis of classical galactosaemia. The enzyme activity has been related to several cell

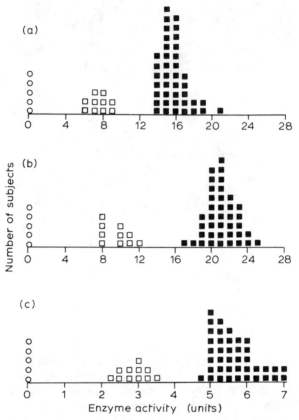

Fig. 5.2 Distribution of red cell activity of galactose-1-phosphate uridyl transferase expressed as μmol substrate converted. (a) Substrate converted h^{-1} g protein^{-1}. (b) Substrate converted h^{-1} g haemoglobin^{-1}. (c) Substrate converted h^{-1} per ml packed red cells. The genotypes are: ○, galactosaemia homozygotes; □, normal/galactosaemia heterozygotes; ■, normal homozygotes.

parameters but, in this case, the ratio of transferase to haemoglobin concentrations gives the best means of differentiating the genotypes. Homozygous normal, homozygous abnormal and heterozygous subjects are clearly distinguished.

There are two main problems with the enzyme method:

(1) The enzyme of interest may not be present, or its deficiency may not be expressed, in biological material which is readily available. It is easy to obtain blood, for enzyme assay in plasma,

leukocytes or erythrocytes, or a small skin biopsy from which cultured fibroblasts may be grown. Apart from this, much more difficult tissue biopsy techniques may be required. Phenylketonuria provides a good example of this problem because phenylalanine hydroxylase, the affected enzyme in this condition, is confined almost entirely to the liver. In most cases it is not considered justifiable to do a liver biopsy to make the diagnosis.

(2) The normal variation of enzyme activity may be so large that it is difficult to distinguish the abnormal individual. Figure 5.3 shows this problem in attempting to diagnose the condition of hypophosphatasia by assaying alkaline phosphatase in cultured amniotic fluid cells. Sometimes a large part of the variation in normal enzyme activity may be methodological in origin. However, it may be that genetic variations in the normal population are the cause.

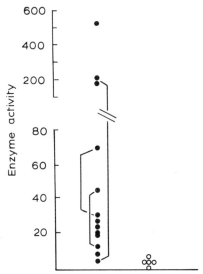

Fig. 5.3 Alkaline phosphatase in cultured amniotic fluid cells. ●, activities in normal pregnancies (linked points indicate assays on duplicate cultures from the same amniotic fluid); ○, results from two pregnancies with an affected fetus.

A good example of low activity mutants extending the normal range, and complicating the diagnosis of the true deficiency, again involves the enzyme transferase. There is a relatively common mutant allele, called the Duarte gene, which produces an enzyme having 40 to 50% of the activity of the usual 'normal' gene. The

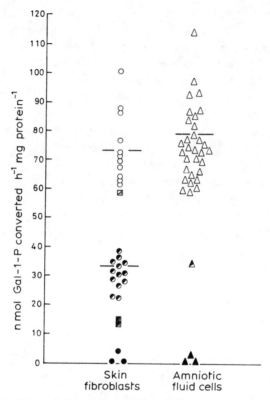

Fig. 5.4 Galactose-l-phosphate uridyl transferase activity in cultured skin fibroblasts and amniotic fluid cells. ○ △ , normal homozygotes; ◐ ▲ , normal/galactosaemia heterozygotes; ● ▲ , galactosaemia homozygotes; ▣ normal/Duarte heterozygotes; ▨ , galactosaemia/Duarte heterozygotes.

transferase activity in cultured skin fibroblasts and amniotic fluid cells from individuals with various genotypes is shown in Fig. 5.4. The results with skin fibroblasts include subjects possessing the Duarte gene. Those who are homozygous for the galactosaemia (transferase 'deficient') gene may have measurable levels of enzyme in fibroblasts, up to 6% of the mean activity for those homozygous for the normal gene. Heterozygotes for the galactosaemia and Duarte gene have as little as 16% of the mean normal level. Mild galactosaemic symptoms have very rarely been described in some of these heterozygotes, particularly during the newborn period, but they are on the whole asymptomatic.

In families in which the Duarte and galactosaemia gene co-exist the differentiation of truly deficient individuals from those who will be clinically normal may be quite exacting. This is certainly a critical decision in prenatal diagnosis, because only homozygous galacto-saemia fetuses should be aborted. The distinction of genotype may be assisted in the case of red cell transferase assay by the use of iso-electric focussing (Fig. 5.5).

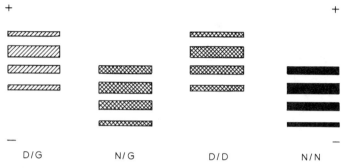

Fig. 5.5 Iso-electric focussing of galactose-1-phosphate uridyl transferase variants. Transferase variants may be distinguished by separating the enzymes on polyacrylamide gels between a pH gradient of 5.0 and 6.5. The galactosaemia variant has no activity and cannot be detected on the gel. The Duarte variant enzyme produces bands with a pI between 5.5 and 5.8; the normal enzyme bands between 5.7 and 6.0. D/G, Duarte/galactosaemia heterozygotes; N/G, normal/galactosaemia heterozygotes; D/D, Duarte homozygotes; N/N, normal homozygotes.

5.2.3 *Metabolite analysis*

Metabolite analysis was the original method of making a diagnosis and remains the most widely used, at least for the initial detection of a disease. However, it should always be remembered that the metabolic changes are secondary consequences of a primary enzyme deficiency and, as such, they may sometimes be unreliable.

The most common method is to demonstrate the accumulation of precursors of the enzyme block in blood plasma or cells, or their increased excretion in the urine (see Fig. 1.2(c)). Unfortunately, this enhanced precursor level may only exist so long as the preceeding compounds continue to prime the pathway.

With regard to the use of abnormal metabolites as a means of diagnosis (Fig. 1.2(d)), it has to be appreciated that their synthesis will usually require specific enzymes. If these enzymes happen not to be present the abnormal metabolites will not be formed, and the diagnosis will be missed.

Since the problems of the use of metabolites are particularly relevant to diagnosis in the newborn, they will be elaborated on in the section on newborn screening.

5.3   Conventional diagnostic procedures

The conventional, and by far the most common, diagnostic situation is that in which a clinician suspects a diagnosis as a result of his observations of a patient's symptoms and signs. His tentative ideas may, or may not, be confirmed by laboratory investigations.

The disadvantage of this procedure is that it often leads to diagnosis being delayed, or even missed completely. This is understandable, because it is impossible for each clinician to have a personal knowledge of hundreds of metabolic diseases which individually are extremely rare. The problem is compounded because a lot of the diseases lack very specific, or characteristic symptoms. The difficulty exists particularly in the diagnosis of inherited metabolic diseases in very ill infants and children. The diagnosis is frequently missed in these circumstances or delayed until a time when irreversible damage has occured, rendering treatment of little value.

It is clear that good laboratory facilities are required to ensure accurate and rapid results once a presumptive diagnosis has been made. In these special circumstances a wide range of samples may be obtained from a patient and the biopsy of muscle, liver or intestine may sometimes be justified in order to make a definitive diagnosis.

5.4   Newborn population screening

5.4.1   Introduction

The advantages of newborn population screening are that it ensures complete and early detection of cases of a specific disease. This is important when an established treatment is available which is particularly successful if started early in life. Phenylketonuria is the disorder which is screened for most widely in the newborn. Screening is normally performed between 6 and 14 days of age and this enables treatment to be introduced by about 3 weeks. In these circumstances, the development of patients appears to proceed absolutely normally and the intellectual development is extremely close to that expected from the family background.

The main disadvantage of newborn screening is the high cost of testing every baby in order to make the diagnosis in a relatively small proportion of the population. The incidence of phenylketonuria is about 1 in 10 000 in most populations, a level which is thought to justify screening; but many diseases are as rare as 1 in 100 000 births. The expansion of screening in different countries depends very much on the relative amount of money which can be spent on health.

5.4.2 Practical aspects

The samples which are fairly readily obtained in large scale newborn screening studies are:

(1) Blood obtained at birth from the umbilical cord and, later, from capillary samples by pricking the heel. For ease of collection and transportation the blood samples may be allowed to soak onto filter paper. Many analyses may now be performed on these dry blood spots.

(2) Urine, which may be collected conveniently by leaving a filter paper inside a nappy.

Nearly all methods for the diagnosis of inherited diseases on newborn samples depend on assaying abnormal levels of metabolites. Galactosaemia, however, may be diagnosed using an assay for transferase which may be done on cord blood or dried blood spot.

Diagnoses using metabolite assays are inherently difficult in the newborn for a number of reasons:

(1) Levels of a precursor, which normally accumulates in the body in a particular enzyme defect, may not be increased at birth because, during intrauterine life, it passes from the fetus, through the placenta, to the maternal circulation and is metabolized. Precursor levels increase only when the baby starts an independent existence and may require the commencement of normal feeding.

Blood phenylalanine levels are normal at birth in phenylketonuric patients but rise to maximum concentrations during the first 2 to 3 weeks of life. Screening for the detection of the condition is rarely performed before the sixth day of life, because if carried out much earlier than this there is a risk of missing the diagnosis.

(2) The increased concentration of precursors, or production of abnormal metabolites, may be dependant on regular feeds and may fluctuate in relation to the timing of feeds. Since vomiting and feeding difficulties are common in the early days of life, and may be a specific feature of some metabolic diseases, the biochemical signs of a condition may be intermittent. It has been shown, for example, that the presence of galactose in urine, an observation which is used frequently to test for galactosaemia, is not a constant feature in all cases of the disease.

(3) The maturation of some enzyme systems may occur only weeks, or months after birth. If the production of the abnormal metabolite characteristic of a particular inherited disease is dependent on one of these late maturing enzymes, the biochemical sign may be absent in the early stages of life.

Phenylketonuria affords a good example of this problem, also. In the mature patient the urinary excretion of phenylpyruvic acid is a good diagnostic sign and was, indeed, the means by which the disease was first discovered. However, when the original newborn screening programmes for phenylketonuria were introduced using a test for phenylpyruvic acid, it was found that as many as half of the cases of the disease were being missed. It became apparent later that this was because a liver transaminase, which converts accumulated phenylalanine to phenylpyruvic acid, was absent from the liver of some infants for many weeks. It was at this stage that blood phenylalanine measurement was introduced as the screening test.

5.5 Prenatal diagnosis

5.5.1 General principles of prenatal diagnosis

Prenatal diagnosis is indicated when there is an established risk of a fetus being affected by a recessively inherited metabolic disorder. The usual intention is to terminate the pregnancy if the fetus is found to be homozygous abnormal for the disease. In this way, parents may elect to have only clinically normal children with respect to the specific disorder they are at risk for. Some 60 or more diseases are amenable to management in this way.

There are important ethical considerations in the practice of prenatal diagnosis. To begin with, there are some people to whom the whole procedure is completely unacceptable on religious or moral grounds. For many, however, prenatal diagnosis and pregnancy termination would be considered for inherited diseases which cause very severe abnormality and for which there is no satisfactory treatment. There are wide variations in attitudes; other parents may wish to prevent the birth of children with even minor degrees of handicap. Against the presumed advantages of prenatal diagnosis, the dangers of the procedure have to be taken into account. Most experts believe that there are small, but finite, risks to the fetus from all the methods used for obtaining the material for the diagnosis, which are described in the next section. These risks range from loss of the fetus, to the birth of a baby with physical defects. Unfortunately these complications are just as likely to affect a baby who does not have the inherited disease.

Legal and personal considerations dictate that termination should be carried out as early as possible in the pregnancy. A target of 20 weeks gestation is usually accepted as the latest time for the result of prenatal diagnosis to be available, but earlier is preferable. It will become apparent that this time factor is critical in determining the best techniques; and the trend is towards methods which are able to provide diagnosis very early in the pregnancy.

Couples are usually found to have a risk of producing children with an inherited metabolic disease following the birth of an affected child. It is imperative to establish a precise diagnosis in the abnormal child, particularly if a prenatal diagnosis is subsequently carried out. Should the wrong disease be suspected and an inappropriate prenatal diagnostic test performed, the result will inevitably be normal. If the opportunity to make a definitive diagnosis on the affected child is missed, the problem may sometimes be overcome by proving that both parents are in the heterozygote range for a specific enzyme defect.

The disadvantage of the above procedure is that an abnormal child has first to be born in order to establish the parental risk. In order to overcome this difficulty there have been experiments in heterozygote detection, to define couples in the population who are at risk for a particular inherited disease before they even contemplate having a family. Providing the genetic counselling and prenatal diagnosis is successful in these couples, it should be possible to prevent the disease completely, apart from the chance of new mutations occurring. This type of heterozygote screening is a workable proposition only in very special circumstances. Firstly it is necessary to have a simple and extremely accurate method for heterozygote detection. Secondly, in order to be economically feasible the disease must have a very high incidence in a well-defined population. Thirdly, the population needs to be extremely well motivated towards the elimination of the particular disease.

The criteria for a successful heterozygote screening programme are likely to be fulfilled for only a few diseases, but the exercise has been tried fairly successfully in one or two instances. The widest application has been in the field of haemoglobin disorders, which are confined to African Negro populations. In the inherited metabolic diseases, Tay Sachs disease is almost exclusively found in Ashkenazie Jews. The people of this race have organized screening programmes to detect heterozygotes for the disease, particularly in the city of New York.

5.5.2 *Sources of fetal material and prenatal diagnosis*

(a) *Chorionic villi*
In the last few years there has been growing interest in the use of chorionic villi for prenatal diagnosis. Chorionic villi are the projections from the developing embryo which implant into the expanding corpus luteum of the mother, later forming the placenta. Small pieces of the villi may be obtained at about 8 to 10 weeks gestation, usually by a transcervical route (Fig. 5.6). It is too early to assess the risks of the procedure, but there are no indications that they are excessively high.

A biopsy of about 10 mg of chorion can be obtained and healthy villi free of maternal contaminating material must be separated from the specimen. Diagnostic tests may be carried out immediately, or the villi may be grown first in tissue culture. Direct testing is attractive since it offers the earliest possible means of prenatal diagnosis.

There are very few examples of the successful use of chorionic villi for prenatal diagnosis by enzyme assay and there is one probable disadvantage to this technique. Quantitation of enzyme activity may be difficult since the amount of intact, really viable, cells which are taken in the assay will be unknown. The best answer to this problem may be to express the activity of the test enzyme in relation to that of

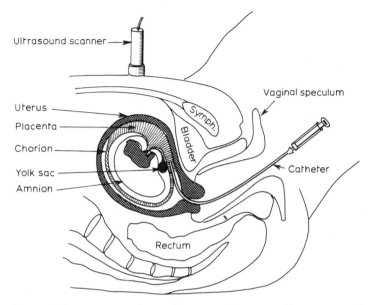

Fig. 5.6 The aspiration of a small biopsy of chorionic villi transcervically.

a suitable reference enzyme. On the other hand chorionic villi may prove to be an excellent source of fetal DNA for a prenatal diagnosis by the DNA polymorphism technique.

(b) Fetal blood

Fetal blood may be obtained by inserting a needle through the mother's abdomen, into the uterine cavity, and aspirating blood from the surface, or fetal side, of the placenta. The disadvantage of this technique is that amniotic fluid is often aspirated as well. A rather more satisfactory method is to insert the needle into the umbilical cord, close to where it is joined to the placenta and where it is in a reasonably stable position. Up to 1.0 ml of uncontaminated fetal blood may be obtained by the latter method.

Fetal blood sampling is the most risky procedure of all those which have been used routinely for prenatal diagnosis. Fetal loss has occurred in about 3% of cases in which the technique has been performed. It has proved important for the prenatal diagnosis of haemoglobin disorders, but hardly any situations arise in the metabolic disease field in which a safer and more acceptable method is not available.

(c) *Amniotic fluid*

Most prenatal diagnoses for inherited metabolic diseases have been performed on amniotic fluid. This is obtained by transabdominal amniocentesis (Fig. 5.7), usually carried out between 14 and 16 weeks gestation. There has been much disagreement about the risk of the procedure. Some consider that it is negligible; others believe that they have shown that there is a small but definite fetal loss, occurring in about 1% of amniocenteses.

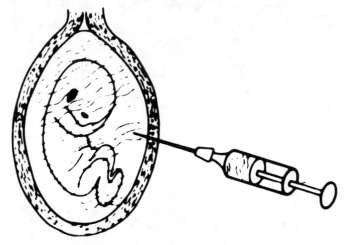

Fig. 5.7 Sampling amniotic fluid from around the fetus approaching transabdominally.

Amniotic fluid is separated by low speed centrifugation into supernatant and sediment. The sediment is composed mainly of cells shed from the skin and other external surfaces of the fetus, but one should beware of possible contamination with maternal cells. The proportion of intact, viable, fetal cells may be as low as 20% of the total material, with the possibility of the remainder discharging their contents into the supernatant fluid.

The component solutes of amniotic fluid supernatant originate from both the mother and the fetus and, as has been mentioned above, from degenerating cells which have been shed by the fetus. In early pregnancy small molecular weight metabolites move freely across permeable membranes into the fluid, from both maternal and fetal circulations. However, starting at about 12 weeks gestation, and increasingly as pregnancy progresses, the fetus has a predominant influence on amniotic fluid composition because of the excretion of fetal urine into the amniotic fluid compartment.

Thus cellular and supernatant composition of amniotic fluid will probably reflect abnormalities in the fetus. Exploitation of the fluid for prenatal diagnosis will be discussed in the last two sections of the book.

5.5.3   Prenatal diagnosis using amniotic fluid supernatant

It was explained in the previous section that, in the second trimester of pregnancy, the amniotic fluid supernatant contains the contents of fetal cells which have 'leaked out' and, also, compounds which have been excreted by the fetal kidney. The enzymes found in the supernatant come mostly from the degenerate cells. If the fetus has an inherited defect involving one of the enzymes normally present in amniotic fluid, it may be possible to make a diagnosis by investigating the defect in the supernatant.

However, simply measuring enzyme activity may be unsatisfactory, because this will depend very much on the extent to which the cells have degenerated. This problem may be overcome if the defective enzyme can be measured as a ratio to a suitable reference izyme. It is then only necessary to assume that the test and reference enzymes leak out of the amniotic fluid cells at the same rate. The method has been used successfully in the diagnosis of Tay Sachs disease, in which the affected enzyme, hexosaminidase A, is measured as a ratio to the activity of its isoenzyme, hexosaminidase B.

Prenatal diagnosis is possible also from the metabolite composition of amniotic fluid. Fetal accumulation of precursors, or formation of abnormal metabolites, consequent upon an enzyme block, may be reflected in the composition of the supernatant fluid. General observations about the limitations of this method of detecting enzyme deficiencies have been discussed and these would certainly apply to fetal diagnosis. Moreover, additional difficulties would be anticipated in prenatal diagnosis. The most important of these arises because of the alternative route of removing compounds in the fetus, through the placenta and the maternal circulation. Maternal metabolism and excretion may completely modify the biochemical expression of an enzyme defect. Reference has been made to the fact that phenylketonuria does not develop until after birth. The other consideration is that the immature fetal kidney may not always be able to excrete some abnormal metabolites into the amniotic fluid,

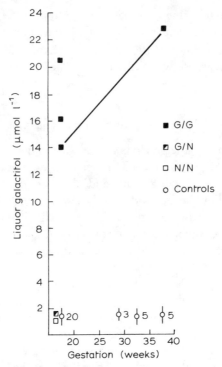

Fig. 5.8 The prenatal detection of galactosaemia by measuring amniotic fluid galactitol. ■, galactitol levels in three pregnancies with a homozygous abnormal fetus (the line links two values obtained at different times in the same pregnancy); ◪, a pregnancy with a fetus which is galactosaemia/normal heterozygose; □, a pregnancy 'at risk' for galactosaemia, but with a homozygous normal fetus; o, pregnancies not known to be 'at risk' for galactosaemia.

although the same compounds are an invariable feature in the urine of adults with a particular disease.

Early experience seemed to suggest that metabolite analysis of amniotic fluid was unreliable as a method of prenatal diagnosis. More recently a number of successful applications of this approach have been described. For example, the level of the metabolite galactitol, which is formed in galactosaemia (Section 4.3.2), can be used to predict the presence of the disease in the fetus (Fig. 5.8). The attraction of a simple analysis of amniotic fluid for prenatal diagnosis is that a result can be available very soon after the amniocentesis has been performed.

5.5.4 Prenatal diagnosis using amniotic fluid cells: tissue culture techniques

The cellular debris obtained from centrifuged amniotic fluid has been used for prenatal diagnosis directly, but it is not recommended. Just as quantitative enzyme measurements are not usually meaningful on the supernatant fluid, similar assays on amniotic fluid cells have their limitations because an indeterminate proportion of the cells have lost their enzymes. The cellular material may be a very useful source of DNA for diagnostic tests, but this approach has not been widely used as yet in the metabolic disease field.

The usual method for using amniotic fluid cells, and by far the most common method of making a prenatal diagnosis at the present time, is to grow them in tissue culture. The objectives of culturing the cells are:

(1) To ensure that the cells used for enzyme assay are intact and viable.

(2) To produce a homogeneous cell line of consistent enzyme composition.

(3) To make a large number of cells should the assay method require them.

Cell cultures are initiated by suspending the centrifuged deposit from the amniotic fluid in a small volume of a nutrient medium which contains, typically, amino acids, lipids, glucose, vitamins, nucleic acids, inorganic ions and fetal calf serum. The medium is maintained at 37°C in an atmosphere of 5% CO_2 in air. The growing cells attach to the bottom of the culture vessel in about 3 or 4 days and, once this has occurred, the medium may be changed every few days in order to stimulate maximum growth. A monolayer of cells will soon cover the base of the flask and at this point the growth is said to be confluent.

The initial, or primary, culture has been used for diagnosis, but has given rise to errors because the clones of cells within it may still be heterogeneous. The principle type of cell is the fibroblast, but it may be of variable enzyme composition at this stage. In addition, epithelial cells may be present, with quite different morphological and enzyme characteristics to the fibroblast and, possibly, maternal cells. Obviously the assay of maternal cells should be completely avoided.

The problem of cell heterogeneity is overcome by sub-culturing

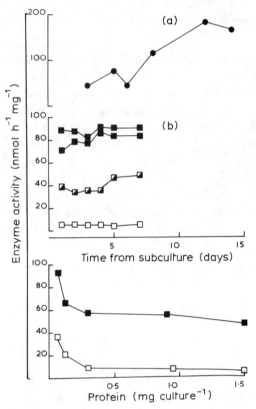

Fig. 5.9 Different patterns of enzyme activity with time in amniotic fluid cell sub-cultures. Enzyme activity is expressed per mg of protein. (a) α-Glucosidase assayed from 3 to 15 days after sub-culture. (b) Galactose-1-phosphate uridyl transferase (expressed as Gal-l-P converted) on days 1 to 7 after sub-culture. ■, homozygous normal cells; ◩, normal/galactosaemia heterozygous cells; □, homozygous galactosaemic cells. (c) Galactose-l-phosphate uridyl transferase (expressed as Gal-1-P converted, with increasing cell growth measured in terms of mg protein culture⁻¹. Symbols are as in (b). Note an apparent difference in (b) and (c) in the changing pattern of transferase activity with increasing cell growth as obtained in two different laboratories.

and growing secondary cultures. The cells of the primary culture are dislodged from the culture vessel by incubating in a solution of trypsin in EDTA, and they are harvested by centrifuging the incubated mixture. Aliquots of the cells are seeded into fresh culture medium to begin a new growth and to reach confluency, usually in 4 to 7 days. In the secondary cultures fibroblasts usually outgrow all other cell lines and a homogeneous product is obtained. Cells for enzyme assay have to be harvested, as previously described, and then disrupted by osmotic shock, sonication or freezing and thawing. Sensitive enzyme assays are used so that as few cells as possible are needed and the results are usually expressed in relation to the protein content of the cell homogenate. Enzyme activity may vary with the age of the cells and, therefore, it is important to study the relationship of enzyme concentration and length of time the cells have been in sub-culture. This is usually a constant characteristic of a given enzyme (Fig. 5.9). It is best to perform the prenatal diagnosis when the enzyme activity is optimal, and not rapidly changing with time.

The technique of prenatal diagnosis with cultured cells has proved very reliable and, at present, is regarded as the reference method. At least 60 diseases may be diagnosed, the limitation to this being the number of enzymes which are normally expressed in fibroblast cells. It has the serious disadvantage that, if the cell growth is slow, or if many cells are necessary for the enzyme assay, the time to achieve a diagnosis may be unacceptably long. The deadline of 20 weeks gestation for a result may be difficult to meet, and this is the main reason that alternative methods are being sought.

Suggestions for further reading and for reference

1 Unfamiliar medical and some scientific words may be looked up quite conveniently in the following medical dictionaries. The first of them gives a very full explanation of each word, often with an illustration. The second is a concise version of the first.

    Stedman's Medical Dictionary, 24th edn (1982) Williams and Wilkins, Baltimore.

    Dorland's Pocket Medical Dictionary, 23rd edn (1982) W.B. Saunders Company, Philadelphia.

2 There are two standard textbooks from which it is possible to obtain a great deal more information about specific diseases. They also have introductory chapters on the history and principles of the inherited metabolic disorders. Although the second of these books is out of date in some respects, the amount of detail it gives is rather less and it may be found more manageable than the first.

    Stanbury, J.B., Wyngaarden, J.B., Fredrickson, D.S., Goldstein, J.L. and Brown, M.S. (eds) (1983) *The Metabolic Basis of Inherited Disease*, 5th edn, McGraw-Hill, New York.

    Bondy, P.K., and Rosenberg, L.E. (eds) (1980) *Metabolic Control and Disease*, 8th edn, W.B. Saunders and Company, Philadelphia.

3 McKusick, V. (1983) *Mendelian Inheritance in Man*, 6th edn, John Hopkins University Press, Baltimore.

    This is an exhaustive and authoritative catalogue of inherited diseases, with and without a known metabolic basis.

4 Harris, H. (1980) *The Principles of Human Biochemical Genetics*, 3rd edn, Elsevier/North Holland Biomedical Press, Amsterdam.

Harris, H. (1982) *Molecular aspects of genetic heterogeneity,* in *Inborn Errors of Metabolism in Humans* (eds F. Cockburn and R. Gitzelmann), MTP Press, Lancaster, pp. 3–12.

Professor Harris was the first person to introduce a modern molecular approach to human biochemical genetics and his book fills in some of the background that was impossible to include in this book. His article in the symposium, 'Inborn Errors of Metabolism in Humans', is a more recent update on the subject of genetic heterogeneity.

5 Emery, A.E.H. (1984) *Introduction to Recombinant DNA,* John Wiley and Sons, Chichester.

Professor Emery's book gives a simple outline of the general principles of DNA techniques and their application in the diagnosis, treatment and prevention of genetic disease.

It also discusses future uses, and problems with the techniques.

6 As stated in the text of this book, the investigation of the haemoglobin disorders has provided the most precise information available on defects in gene expression in humans. The following references are recent reviews of the polymorphism occurring in and around the globin genes and the molecular mechanisms responsible for the thalassaemias.

Higgs, D.R. and Weatherall, D.J. (1983) Alpha-Thalassaemia *Curr. Top. Haematol.,* **4**, 37–97.

Orkin, S.H., Antonarakis, S.E. and Kazazian, H.H. (1983) Polymorphism and molecular pathology of the human beta-globin gene. *Prog. Haematol.,* **13**, 49–73.

7 Holton, J.B. (1983) Prenatal diagnosis in inherited metabolic disease, neural tube defects and lung maturity, in *Scientific Foundations of Clinical Biochemistry in Clinical Practice,* (eds D.L. Williams and V. Marks), William Heinemann Medical Books Ltd., London, pp. 663–681.

This is a detailed account of the general principles underlying the practice of prenatal diagnosis and of the rather specialized techniques employed.

Index

Acatalasia 42
N-Acetylhexosaminidase 35
  A and B forms 35
  deficiencies 34
  protein activator 36
  sub-unit gene loci 35
Acidosis, in methylmalonic
    aciduria 18
Acid phosphatase, red cell 25
  electrophoresis 26
Acute intermittent porphyria 67
Adenosyl biotin 19
Adenosyl cobalamin 19, 36, 58
Adenylate cyclase 72
Albinism 2, 56
Albumin 8
Alkaline phosphatase deficiency 79
Alkapton 1
Alkaptonuria 1
Amino acid transport
  brain 61
  intestine 69
  renal tubule 69, 70
γ-Aminobutyric acid synthesis 65
γ-Aminolaevulinic acid
    synthetase 67
Amniocentesis 88
Amniotic fluid 88
  cell culture 91
  supernatant 88, 89
α_1-Antitrypsin
  deficiency 49
  structure 49
Apoenzyme-cofactor binding 13,
  16
Apoenzyme-substrate binding 13,
  15
Arginase 14

Argininosuccinase 14
Argininosuccinic acid
  synthetase 14
  deficiency 14, 31
Aspartyl transcarbamylase 22
Autosomal dominant
  inheritance 5, 45
  genotype of offspring in 5
Autosomal recessive inheritance 4
  genotype of offspring in 5

Beadle and Tatum 4

Cap group, RNA 10
Carbamyl phosphate synthetase 14
Cataracts 64
Catecholamine synthesis 65
Cathepsin 55
C_1-esterase inhibitor 8
Chorionic villus 86
  biopsy 87
Chromosome
  5 35
  11 11
  15 35
  16 11
Citrullinaemia 14
Coagulation factors 8
Coding regions, gene 9
Complement 8
CRM, see Cross reacting material
Cross reacting material
  methylmalonyl-CoA mutase 36
Cystathioninase 16, 17
  deficiency 16
  heterogeneity 17
Cystathionine-β-synthetase 17
  deficiency 19, 42

Cystathioninuria 16
Cystine 2, 71
Cystinuria 2, 71

Dent and Rose 7
Diagnosis 74
Dibucaine 15
Dibucaine number 16
Diet
   in phenylketonuria 32, 60
   affecting clinical expression 46
Dihydroorotase 22
Dihydroorotic acid
   dehydrogenase 22
Distribution defects 49
DNA polymorphisms 75
   use in diagnosis 75, 76, 87
DNA probe 75, 76

Elastase 50
Endocytosis 37, 72
Enzyme instability 19, 40
Eumelanin 56, 57
Exons 9, 10
Expression of genes, X
   chromosome 6

Favism 20
Feedback control 66
Fetal blood sampling 87
Fibroblast cells 91, 92
   in argininosuccinic acid
      synthetase deficiency 14
Følling 32

Galactitol
   cataract formation 64
   prenatal diagnosis
      galactosaemia 90
Galactokinase 41
   deficiency 61
Galactosaemia, *see* Galactose-l-
   phosphate uridyl transferase
   deficiency
Galactose, metabolic pathways 41

Galactose-l-phosphate 61
Galactose-l-phosphate uridyl
   transferase 41
   deficiency 61, 77, 78
   diagnostic use 77, 78, 80, 83, 84,
      92
   Duarte variant 79, 80, 81
   prenatal diagnostic use 90, 92
Garrod 1
Gaussian distribution 25
Gene
   diagnostic use 75
   dosage 25, 41
   expression, mechanism of 10
   probe, *see* DNA probe
   transcription 10
Glucose-6-phosphatase deficiency,
      see Glycogen storage disease
      Type 1.
Glucose-6-phosphate
   dehydrogenase
   deficiency 20, 21
   leukocyte 40
   variant forms
      A 28
      Athens 28
      B 28
      Canton 28
      Hektoen 28
      Mediterranean 20, 21
      Negro 20, 21
α-Glucosidase 92
Glutathione reductase 20
Glycogen storage disease
   Type 1, glucose-6-phosphatase
      deficiency 56
   Type V, muscle phosphorylase
      deficiency 39
   Type VI, liver phosphorylase
      deficiency 39
GM_2-gangliosidosis 35, 36
Growth hormone 8
Growth retardation 21, 51, 71

Haem biosynthesis 67

Haemoglobin disorders 8, 10, 11,
    31, 86, 87
  Hb Barts hydrops foetalis 11
  Hb S 11
Haemolytic anaemia 20, 32, 40
Hartnup disease 71
Heterozygote 4
  clinical expression 44
Hexokinase 20
Histidinaemia 29, 42
L-Histidine ammonia lyase 29
Homocystinuria 19, 46
Homogentisic acid 1
Homozygote 4
Hormone receptors 72
Hurler disease 51
Hydroxy cobalamin 36
5-Hydroxytryptamine synthesis 65
Hypoglycaemia 18
Hypophosphatasia 79

I-cell disease 51
Identity markers 55
α-L-Iduronidase 52, 53
Imino-glycinuria 72
Immunoglobulins 8
Infection and clinical expression 47
Insulin 8
Intergenic DNA 9, 11
Intervening sequences 9, 11
Introns 9, 10
IVS, *see* Intervening sequences

α-Ketoglutarate: glyoxylate
    carboligase 64

Leaky mutations 56
Lipoproteins 8
Low density lipoprotein 72
Lyon hypothesis 6, 45
Lyonization 7
Lysosomal storage diseases 51

Megaloblastic anaemia 21
Melanins 2, 56

Membrane transport defects 7, 68
Mental retardation 14, 16, 30, 32,
    46, 51
Messenger RNA 10
Methyl cobalamin 37
Methylmalonic aciduria 18, 36, 58,
    60
Methylmalonyl-CoA mutase 18,
    19, 36
Methylmalonyl-CoA racemase 18
Mucopolysaccharidoses 51
Multilocus enzymes 39
Multiple allelism 30
Multiple enzymes 38
Multiple gene loci 34
Myelin formation 60, 61

Newborn screening 82
Nonsense mutations 12
Normal distribution 25

One gene – one enzyme
    hypothesis 4
Ornithine transcarbamylase 14
  deficiency 45
Orotic acid 21
Orotic aciduria 21
Orotidine-5′-monophosphate
    decarboxylase 22
Orotidine-5′-monophosphate
    pyrophosphorylase 22
Oxalate
  plasma and urine 63
  synthetic pathways 64
Oxaluria 63

Parathyroid hormone 72, 73
Pentose phosphate pathway 20
Pentosuria 1
Phenylalanine-4-hydroxylase 32,
    79
Phenylalanine, metabolic
    pathways 33
Phenylketonuria 32, 46, 47, 56
  atypical 32, 33

diagnosis 79, 84
heterozygote 44
pathogenesis 60, 64, 65
Pheomelanin 56, 57
Phosphofructokinase
    deficiency 39
    isoenzymes 40
6-Phosphogluconate
    dehydrogenase 20
Phosphorylase deficiency, *see*
    Glycogen storage disease Types
    V and VI
PKU, *see* Phenylketonuria
Placental sulphatase 7
Plasma cholinesterase 15
Point mutation 11
Porphobilinogen 67, 68
Porphobilinogen deaminase 67
Porphyrias 67
Precursor RNA 10
Prenatal diagnosis 84
Processed RNA 10
Propionyl-CoA carboxylase 18
    adenosyl cobalamin cofactor 19
Pseudocholinesterase, *see* Plasma
    cholinesterase
Pseudohypoparathyroidism 73
Pi type, α_1 antitrypsin 49
Pyridoxal-5-phosphate 16, 19
Pyrophosphorylase 41
Pyruvate kinase, red cell,
    deficiency 32

Restriction endonuclease 75
Restriction fragment length
    polymorphisms 76
mRNA, *see* Messenger RNA

Sandhoff disease 34
Scoline sensitivity, *see*
    Succinylcholine sensitivity

Sickle cell disease 11
Spacer DNA 9
Sphingolipids 35, 51
Steroid sulphatase 7
Succinylcholine sensitivity 15, 16

Tay Sachs disease 34, 86
Thalassaemia 11
Thyroid gland 58, 59
Thyroxin synthesis 58, 59
Tissue culture 91
Transcobalamin 37
Transcription 10
Translation 10
Triplet code 11
Tyrosinase 57

Urea cycle 14
Uridine diphosphate-N-
    acetylglucosamine 56
Uridine diphosphate galactose 61
Uridine diphosphate galactose-4-
    epimerase deficiency 40, 61
Uridine-5-monophosphate
    synthesis 22
Uroporphyrinogen synthase, *see*
    Porphobilinogen deaminase

Vitamin
    B_6 16, 19
    B_{12} 19, 36
Von Gierke's disease, *see* Glycogen
    storage disease Type I

Watson-Crick 9

X-chromosome 5
X-linked inheritance
    dominant 7
    recessive 5, 6, 45
Xylulose 1